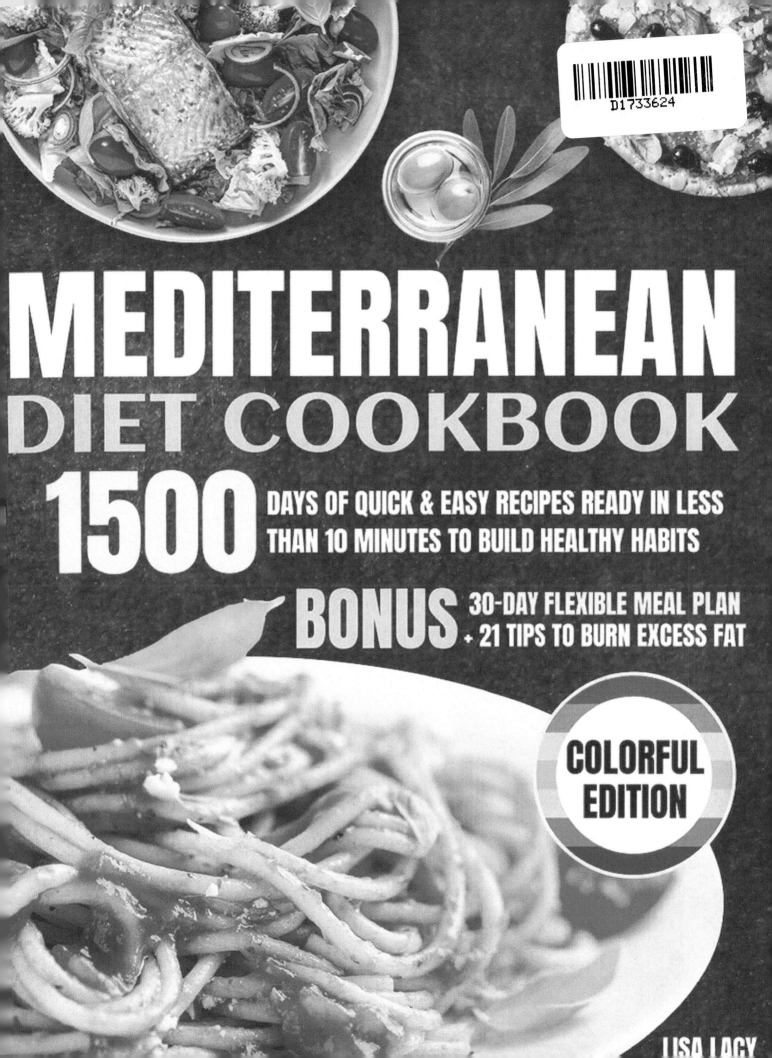

MEDITERRANEAN
DIET COOKBOOK

1500
DAYS OF QUICK & EASY RECIPES READY IN LESS THAN 10 MINUTES TO BUILD HEALTHY HABITS

BONUS 30-DAY FLEXIBLE MEAL PLAN + 21 TIPS TO BURN EXCESS FAT

COLORFUL EDITION

LISA LACY

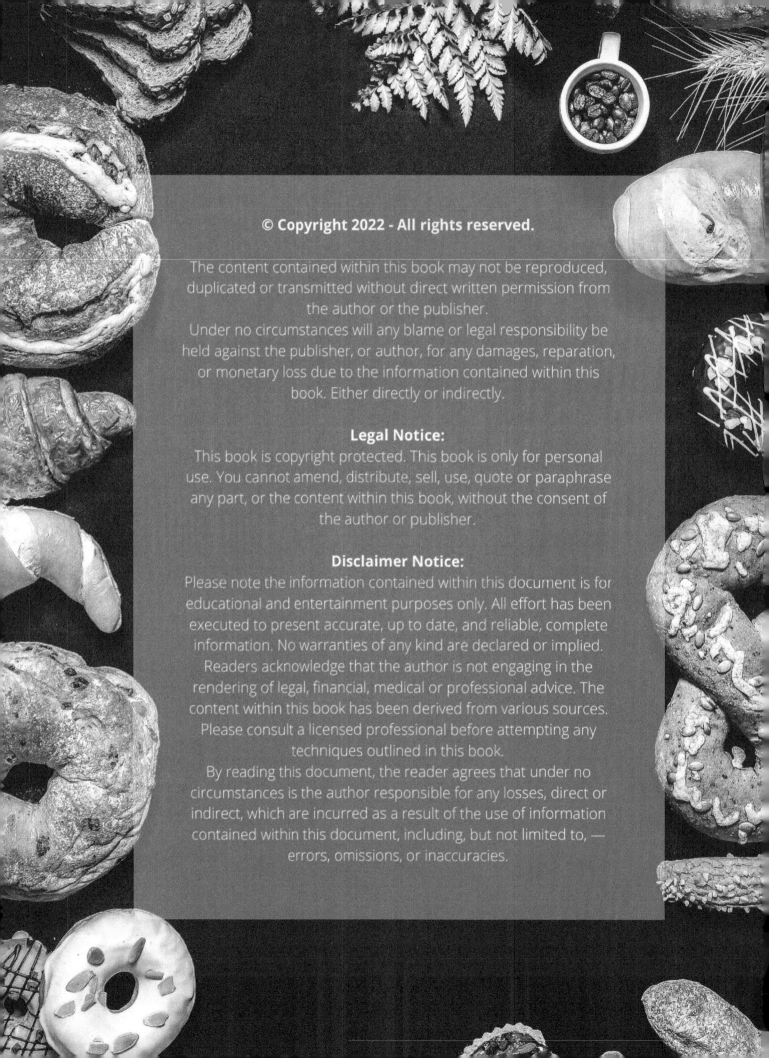

Table of Contents

Introduction

The Mediterranean diet is the best-known in the world. It is a balanced diet based on the intake of fresh and healthy foods, capable of bringing health and well-being to the entire body. At the base of the Mediterranean diet, there are ancient origins that link it to the food origins of the countries bordering the Mediterranean Sea basin.

The first scholar who gave international visibility to the Mediterranean Diet was Ancel Keys, an American biologist and physiologist. Keys contributed to the consolidation of the expression Mediterranean Diet and gave medical and scientific dignity to this expression, codifying the characteristics of the diet. Through a large survey called the "Seven Countries Study," Keys focused on the relationship between the diet of Mediterranean countries and statistics on cardiovascular diseases. The study, considered a milestone in the science of nutrition, shows that the cause of the better health conditions of citizens of Mediterranean countries, especially regarding cardiovascular diseases, is precisely nutrition.

Keys also studied the components of these eating habits and popularized the Mediterranean Diet all over the world, hoping above all that his fellow Americans would change their eating habits to conform to the Mediterranean ones, to improve the general health conditions of the population.

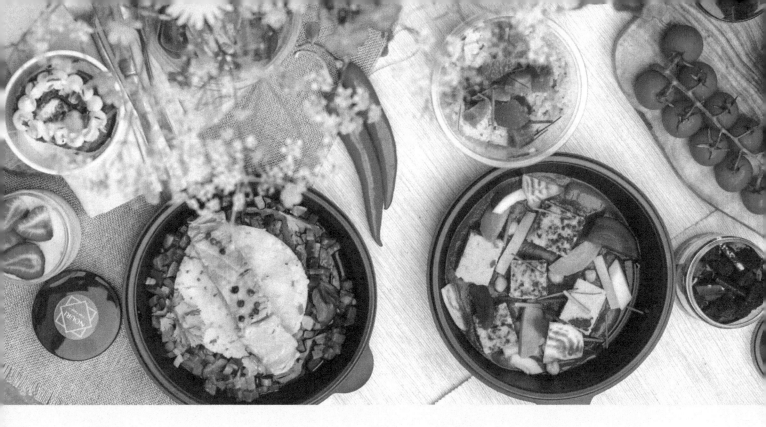

Chapter 1: What Is the Mediterranean Diet

The Mediterranean diet, as we said, is a food style that is based on the culinary tradition of the counries bordering the Mediterranean Sea, such as Spain, Italy, France, Greece, and countries belonging to North Africa, such as Morocco, Libya, and Tunisia.

From the study initiated by Ancel Keys, many other researchers, doing various studies on the eating habits of these countries, have shown that people who followed this dietary style were exceptionally healthy and were at low risk of contracting chronic diseases.

From these studies, it emerged that the Mediterranean diet is very useful not only in promoting weight loss and therefore in combating overweight and obesity, but it is also essential to prevent diseases of the cardiovascular system, such as heart attacks or strokes, or metabolic diseases such as, for example, type 2 diabetes.

For all these reasons, the Mediterranean diet is usually recommended and encouraged in all those cases that involve losing excessive weight or for those who want to improve or prevent certain diseases.

The Mediterranean diet is mainly based on a balanced supply of macronutrients. The largest share of the daily calorie intake must come from carbohydrates ranging from 45–60%. The second share is given by fats ranging from 20–35% and finally proteins which are between 10 and 12%.

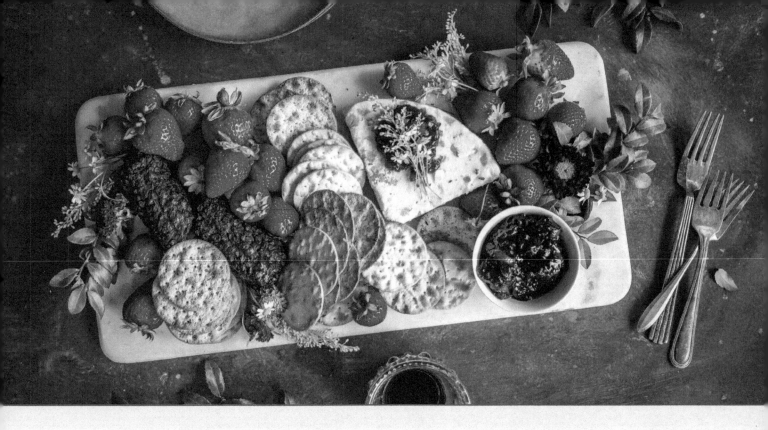

Chapter 2: 10 Benefits of the Mediterranean Diet

The Mediterranean diet is associated with a long list of benefits not only in terms of physical but also mental health.

The beneficial effects of the Mediterranean diet are linked to many factors, such as the richness of foods with a low glycemic index and low-calorie density, which help maintain a healthy weight and ensure a high intake of fiber that protects against the onset of many diseases of the type chronic.

The Mediterranean diet is also characterized by foods that have a low-fat content and are mostly unsaturated, and a high intake of antioxidants, which counteract the effects of free radicals.

Below you will find 10 benefits that the Mediterranean diet brings to the body.

Benefit Number 1: Improves Heart Health

The first benefit that scholars have paid more attention to is certainly the fact that the Mediterranean diet improves heart health. During the research, it was noted that people who followed a Mediterranean-type diet had a lower risk of heart attacks or strokes than those who followed diets based on excessive use of fat or with a total imbalance of all macronutrients.

In addition, many of the foods used in the diet and especially the reduction of sodium intake as a base condiment favors the regulation of blood pressure.

Benefit Number 2: Improves Brain Function

The Mediterranean diet brings enormous benefits to the proper functioning of the brain and above all, it can prevent and protect against cognitive decline.

Some studies have shown that the Mediterranean diet has favored the improvement of cognitive functions by preventing and delaying brain diseases such as dementia, cognitive decline, and Alzheimer's disease.

Another study conducted on healthy seniors showed that the Mediterranean diet had improved cognitive function, memory, and attention span in these subjects.

Benefit Number 3: It Helps Prevent the Onset of Some Cancers

The benefits of the Mediterranean diet also extend to the prevention of some cancers, including breast, colorectal, prostate, stomach, and liver cancers.

The merit is the richness of foods high in antioxidants, which counteract cellular degeneration caused by free radicals, and the low content of highly fatty foods.

In addition, the high fiber content improves intestinal transit, ensuring that potentially dangerous substances do not remain in contact with the walls of the intestine for too long.

Benefit Number 4: Helps Fight Overweight and Obesity

The Mediterranean diet is also very useful if you want to lose a lot of weight and regain your ideal physical shape.

This is because it is rich in fiber, which helps to absorb excess sugars, is low in oxygenated and saturated fats, and above all most of the foods that are part of this diet are low in calories.

Furthermore, if the weight to lose is excessive, simply reduce the amount of carbohydrates from cereals and increase the intake of fruit and especially green leafy vegetables.

Furthermore, the Mediterranean diet will not only help you lose weight, but it will do it healthily. In fact, unlike diets that make you lose weight quickly but just as quickly get you back, this diet will promote steady and gradual weight loss and the benefits will go on for a long time, even when you resume eating normally.

Benefit Number 5: It Is Beneficial and Healthy for Pregnant Women

Being a diet based more on quality than the quantity of foods, the Mediterranean diet is recommended for pregnant women to keep both the woman and the child in good health. This will help to contain the weight gain of the pregnant woman, also protecting her from the risk of contracting metabolic diseases, including gestational diabetes, which can have serious effects on both the woman and the baby.

Furthermore, it is useful for women who are already pregnant with persistent obesity problems, chronic hypertension, and high cholesterol levels.

Benefit Number 6: It Prevents the Risk of Preeclampsia

According to a recent study, it was found that the Mediterranean diet helps prevent the risk of preeclampsia in pregnant women. Preeclampsia is a serious pregnancy complication because it can also lead to the death of the woman.

The study, which was published in the Journal of the American Heart Association, showed that women who followed a Mediterranean diet had reduced the risk of developing preeclampsia during pregnancy by 20%.

The reduced risk is because the Mediterranean diet helps to improve not only oxidative stress but also improves the vascular function of the placenta by making beneficial changes at the metabolic level.

Benefit Number 7: Reduces the Risk of Type 2 Diabetes

The Mediterranean diet is not only useful as a preventative against type 2 diabetes but is also useful in managing the symptoms associated with diabetes.

The advantages of the Mediterranean diet do not only concern a more effective control of blood sugar, but also have a beneficial effect on weight and on the control of fats that accumulate in the liver and blood.

Benefit Number 8: The Mediterranean Diet Reduces Gastroesophageal Reflux

Recent studies conducted by the Feinstein Institute for Medical Research at Northwell Health, and New York Medical College have shown that low-fat diets based on the consumption of fruits and vegetables, just like the Mediterranean diet, reduce gastric reflux by avoiding the use of drugs.

Benefit Number 9: Helps Prevent Kidney Disease

A series of studies conducted on patients with kidney problems have shown that olive oil, which is the basis of the Mediterranean diet, can prevent and counteract the onset of kidney damage.

The study showed that the polyphenols contained in the olive leaves, but also in the olive oil itself, counteract and slow down the progression of some diseases that cause kidney damage. In particular, the polyphenols contained in the leaves and olive oil reduce the growth of kidney cysts by 30–40%.

Benefit Number 10: Reduces Nervous Stress and Helps You Live Better

Stress not only has negative effects on work and personal relationships, but it also increases the risk of many chronic conditions, such as heart disease and Alzheimer's disease.

According to a new study by researchers at Wake Forest School of Medicine, part of Wake Forest Baptist Health, the Mediterranean diet ca reduce the physiological effects of stress and promote healthy aging.

The study showed that the Mediterranean diet promotes greater resistance to stress and a faster recovery after the end of the state of stress.

The results of the study, therefore, suggest that adopting a Mediterranean-type diet can provide a relatively simple and convenient intervention to reduce the negative impact of psychological stress on health and delay the aging of the nervous system.

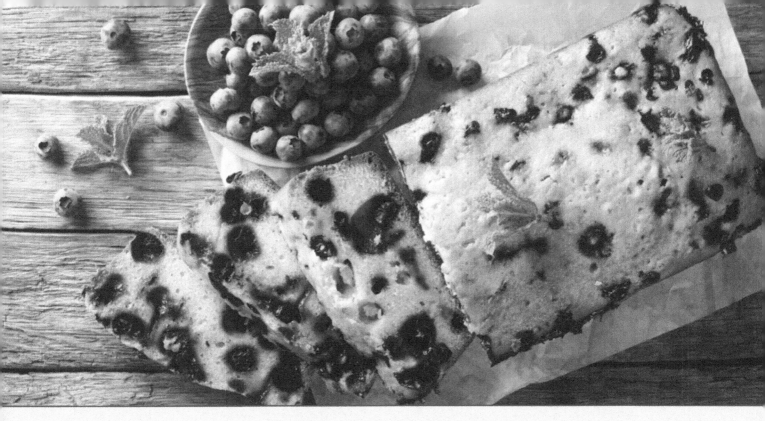

Chapter 3: Shopping List

I t is a bit complicated to establish precisely which food to be included in the Mediterranean diet by the fact that the foods vary according to the countries that fall within the Mediterranean basin.

The basic line of the diet, however, involves the daily consumption of fresh, healthy foods such as fruits and vegetables, which are high in whole carbohydrates and low in protein and fat.

As for the foods to be abolished or taken in moderation, there are all foods containing high amounts of sugars, trans fats, over-processed vegetable oil such as seed oils, over-processed meats with high amounts of fat such as sausage, frankfurters, and cured meats.

The diet also provides for the abolition of all fizzy drinks, too sugary and especially alcohol. Even if the diet includes moderate doses of wine, remember that this is not the norm, that a maximum of one glass of wine is allowed and only once a day for lunch or dinner.

Below you will find a list of products that should not be missing in your pantry if you want to follow this type of diet.

Vegetables	• Tomatoes • Broccoli • Onions • Cabbages • Carrots • Lettuce • Cauliflowers • Spinach • Cucumbers • Turnips • Peppers • Eggplants • Zucchini • Pumpkin
Fruits	• Apples • Bananas • Oranges • Pears • Berries • Strawberries • Grape • Dates • Figs • Melons • Peaches • Cherries • Lemon • Apricot • Kiwi • Almonds • Pistachios • Walnuts • Peanuts
Pasta, rice, grains, amides	• All kinds of legumes • Pasta, preferably wholemeal • Rice, preferably wholemeal

	• Bread, preferably wholemeal • Potatoes
Fish and seafood	• Salmon • Tuna • Sea bream • Sea bass • Cod • Mackerel • Shrimps • Octopus • Squid • Calamari • All kind of mollusks
Meat	• Chicken • Turkey • Beef • Eggs
Dairy	• Milk • Yogurt • Fresh cheese
Sauces and toppings	• Garlic • All kinds of aromatic herbs • Olive oil

Breakfast and Little Dishes

Recipes

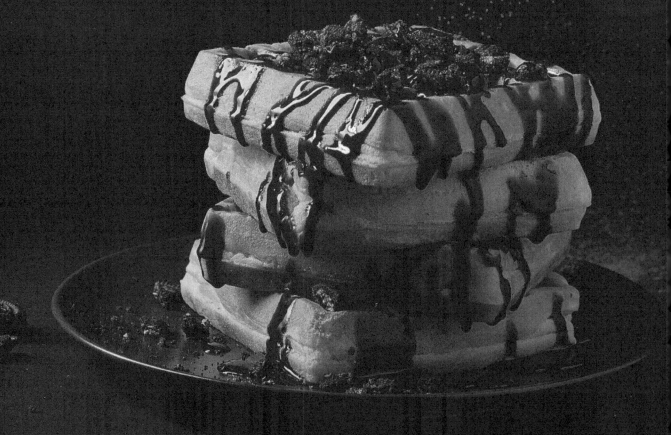

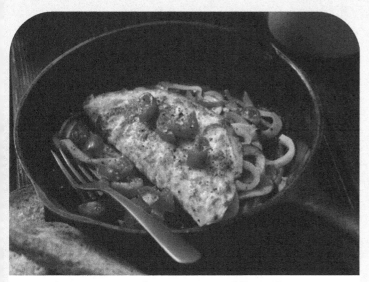

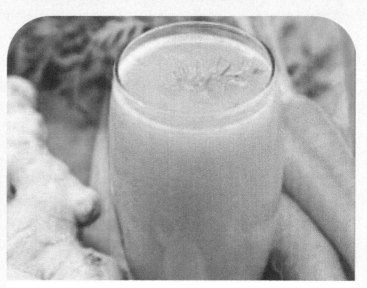

Andalusian Omelette (Spain)

Apricot Smoothie (Italy)

Preparation time: 20 minutes
Cooking time: 20 minutes
Servings: 4
Calories for serving: 173

Preparation time: 20 minutes
Servings: 4
Calories for serving: 132

Macronutrients

Macronutrients

- Carbs: 6 g
- Proteins: 14 g
- Fat: 13 g

- Carbs: 15 g
- Proteins: 3 g
- Fat: 1 g

Ingredients

Ingredients

- 6 eggs
- 1 yellow pepper
- 1 red pepper
- 1.7 oz cooked ham
- Dried oregano to taste
- Olive oil to taste
- Salt and pepper to taste

- 28.2 oz ripe apricots
- 4 tsp honey
- 4 cup unsweetened almond milk
- 16 ice cubes

Directions

Directions

1. Wash the peppers, place them in the oven and cook them at 392°F for 20 minutes. After 20 minutes, take them out of the oven, let them cool and then peel them and cut them into thin strips.

1. Wash the apricots, cut them in half, remove the stone, and put them in the glass of the blender.

2. Break the eggs into a bowl. Add salt, pepper, and oregano and mix with a fork. Then add the peppers, and the ham and mix again.

2. Add the honey, almond milk, and ice.

3. Operate the blender and blend until you get a thick and homogeneous mixture.

3. Heat a little oil in a non-stick pan and then pour the mixture inside. Cook for 3 minutes on each side, then turn off.

4. Put the smoothie in the glasses and serve.

4. Divide the omelet into 4 parts, put it on serving plates and serve.

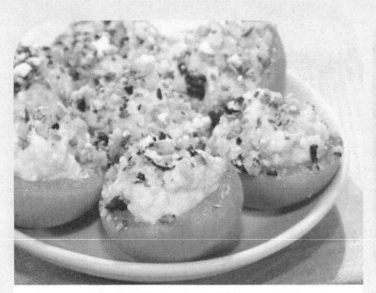

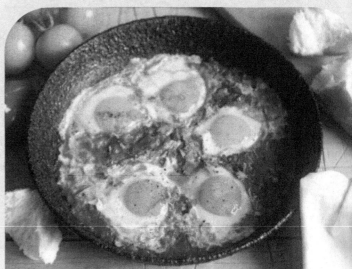

Apricots Stuffed with Tuna (Italy)

Preparation time: 20 minutes
Servings: 4
Calories for serving: 100

Macronutrients

- Carbs: 6 g
- Proteins: 10 g
- Fat: 2 g

Ingredients

- 4 apricots
- 2.8 oz drained canned tuna
- 1.7 oz fresh spreadable cheese
- Chopped rosemary to taste
- Salt and pepper to taste

Directions

1. Put the tuna in a bowl and chop it with a fork. Add the fresh cheese and mix well.
2. Now add salt, pepper, and rosemary and mix again.
3. Wash the apricots, then cut them in half. Remove the stone and season the two parts with the tuna and cheese mixture.
4. Now put the apricots on the serving plates and serve.

Avgà Me Domata, Eggs with Tomato (Greece)

Preparation time: 20 minutes
Cooking time: 15 minutes
Servings: 4
Calories for serving: 184

Macronutrients

- Carbs: 8 g
- Proteins: 6 g
- Fat: 9 g

Ingredients

- 8 eggs
- 4 tomatoes
- Salt and pepper to taste
- Olive oil to taste

Directions

1. Wash the tomatoes, peel them, and then cut them into thin slices. Pour a drizzle of oil into a pan and, when it is hot, add the tomatoes. Season with salt and pepper and cook for 5 minutes.
2. Break the eggs into a bowl and add a little salt and pepper. Beat them well with a fork and then pour them into the saucepan, on top of the tomatoes.
3. Lower the heat and cook for 5 minutes, pricking the mixture with a fork in several places to make it cook better. After 5 minutes, turn the omelet and continue cooking for another 5 minutes.
4. Once cooked, divide the omelet into 4 parts, put it on serving plates, and serve.

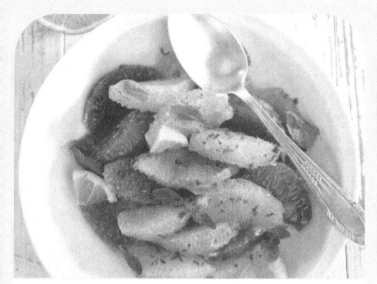

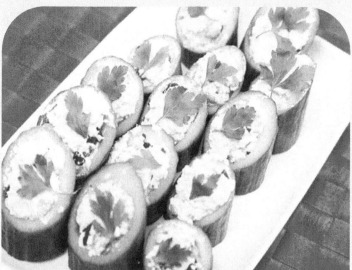

Citrus Fruit Salad with Cinnamon Yogurt (Italy)

Preparation time: 20 minutes + 30 minutes to rest
Servings: 4
Calories for serving: 180

Macronutrients

- Carbs: 32 g
- Proteins: 8 g
- Fat: 8 g

Ingredients

- 2 cups Greek yogurt
- 2 oranges
- 1 pink grapefruit
- 1 grapefruit
- 1 cedar
- 1 lime
- 1 tbsp honey
- 1 tsp cinnamon
- ½ tsp ginger powder

Directions

1. Peel the two types of grapefruit, oranges, and cedar; leave the wedges whole, or cut them into small pieces if they are large and collect them in a bowl.
2. Squeeze the lime, put the juice in a bowl, and add the honey. Mix until you get a homogeneous emulsion. Pour the emulsion over the citrus fruits and mix gently with a wooden spoon to distribute it evenly and flavor the fruit well. Cover the cup with cling film and let it rest in the fridge for 30 minutes.
3. After 30 minutes, take the fruit salad from the fridge and divide it into 4 cups. Put the yogurt in a bowl, add the cinnamon and mix well. Sprinkle the fruit salad with yogurt and serve.

Cucumbers with Fresh Cheese and Cherry Tomatoes (Italy)

Preparation time: 20 minutes
Cooking time: 10 minutes
Servings: 4
Calories for serving: 151

Macronutrients

- Carbs: 7 g
- Proteins: 11 g
- Fat: 12 g

Ingredients

- 2 cucumbers
- 5.2 oz fresh spreadable cheese
- 6 cherry tomatoes
- Dried oregano to taste
- Olive oil to taste
- Salt and pepper to taste

Directions

1. Wash and dry cherry tomatoes, cut them in half, and place them on a baking tray lined with parchment paper. Season with oil, salt, and pepper and put in the oven. Cook at 392°F for 10 minutes.
2. Wash the cucumbers and peel them with a potato peeler. Remove the two ends of each cucumber and cut them into thick slices. Then place the cucumbers on a serving dish.
3. Put the fresh cheese in a bowl and knead it with a fork. Transfer it to a pastry bag with a rather wide opening tip and create small tufts of fresh cheese on each slice of cucumber.
4. Take the cherry tomatoes and put half on each cucumber. Sprinkle with dried oregano and serve.

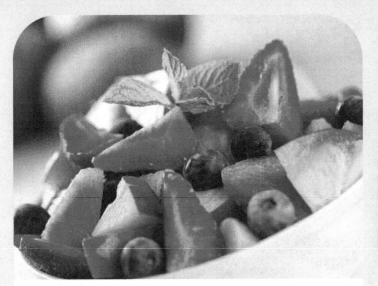

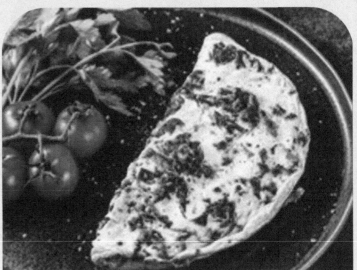

Macedonia with Mint (Italy)

Preparation time: 25 minutes + 2 hours to rest
Servings: 4
Calories for serving: 120

Macronutrients

- Carbs: 27 g
- Proteins: 1 g
- Fat: 0 g

Ingredients

- 1 melon
- 4 peaches
- 5.2 oz raspberries
- 5.2 oz strawberries
- 1 glass orange juice
- 2 tbsp sugar
- 1 bunch fresh mint

Directions

1. Peel the melon, remove the seeds and filaments, and then cut the pulp into cubes.
2. Peel the peaches, remove the stone, and then cut them into wedges. Wash the strawberries, dry them, and then cut them in half. Wash and dry the raspberries.
3. Put the fruit in a bowl. Sprinkle with the sugar and orange juice and mix gently. Put the bowl in the fridge and let it rest for 2 hours.

4. After 2 hours, put the fruit salad in 4 cups, add the washed and dried mint leaves, and serve.

Omelet with Aromatic Herbs (France)

Preparation time: 10 minutes

Cooking time: 10 minutes

Servings: 4

Calories for serving: 184

Macronutrients

- Carbs: 2 g
- Proteins: 8 g
- Fat: 6 g

Ingredients

- 6 eggs
- Chopped parsley to taste
- 1 tbsp chopped chives
- 1 tbsp chopped tarragon
- 1 tbsp chopped chervil
- Salt and pepper to taste
- Olive oil to taste

Directions

1. Break the eggs into a bowl and beat them vigorously with a fork.
2. Add salt, pepper, and herbs and mix again.
3. Heat a little oil in a pan and then pour a little of the mixture. Cook for 2 minutes on each side. Repeat the operation with the rest of the batter until you have made a total of 4 omelets.
4. When all the omelets are cooked, place them on the plates and serve.

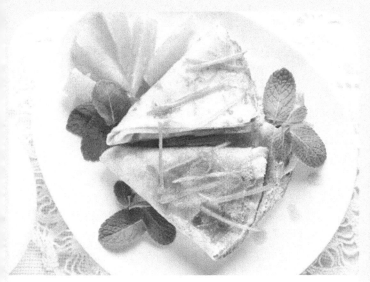

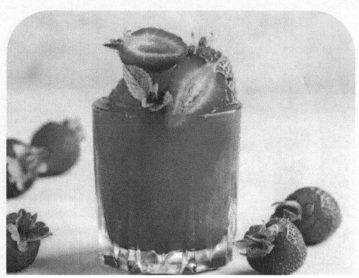

Orange Omelette (France)

Preparation time: 20 minutes
Cooking time: 20 minutes
Servings: 4
Calories for serving: 195

Macronutrients

- Carbs: 15 g
- Proteins: 8 g
- Fat: 10 g

Ingredients

- 4 eggs
- 1 orange
- 3 tbsp sugar
- 2 tbsp butter
- 2 tbsp orange marmalade

Directions

1. Break the eggs and separate the yolks from the whites. Beat the egg whites until stiff.

2. Put the sugar in the bowl with the egg yolks and whip them with an electric mixer until you get a light and fluffy mixture. Incorporate the egg whites into the yolks, mixing from bottom to top.

3. Melt the butter in a baking dish and gently pour in the egg mixture. Place the baking dish in the oven and cook at 302°F for 10 minutes.

4. Meanwhile, put the jam in a saucepan with the juice and orange peel cut into very thin fillets. Heat for 10 minutes, stirring constantly, and then turn off.

5. Once cooked, remove the baking dish from the oven. Put the orange mixture on top of the omelet, cut it into 4 parts, put it on plates, and serve.

Red Fruit Smoothie with Basil (Italy)

Servings: 4

Calories for serving: 138

Macronutrients

- Carbs: 21 g
- Proteins: 6 g
- Fat: 4 g

Ingredients

- 17.6 oz strawberries
- 10.5 oz cherries
- 8.4 oz raspberries
- 7 oz Greek strawberry yogurt
- 1 tbsp chopped basil

Directions

1. Wash the strawberries, cherries, and raspberries and then dry them.
2. Remove the cherry stone and place them in the blender glass.
3. Add the raspberries, strawberries, yogurt, and basil. Operate the blender and blend until you get a creamy and homogeneous mixture.
4. Now pour the smoothie into 4 glasses and serve.

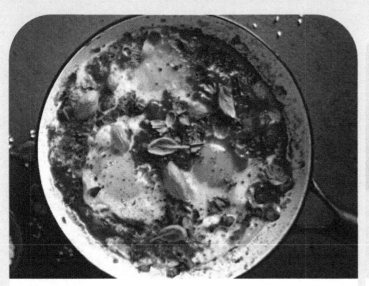

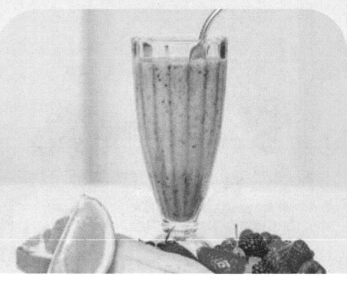

Shakshuka (Israel)

Preparation time: 25 minutes

Cooking time: 20 minutes

Servings: 4

Calories for serving: 271

Macronutrients

- Carbs: 20 g
- Proteins: 12 g
- Fat: 8 g

Ingredients

- 2 onions
- 2 red peppers
- 10 ripe red tomatoes
- 8 eggs
- Salt and pepper to taste
- Paprika to taste
- Cumin powder to taste
- Chopped parsley to taste

Directions

1. Wash the peppers and then cut them into cubes. Wash the tomatoes and cut them into cubes.
2. Peel the onions, chop them, and brown them in a fairly large pan with a little hot olive oil. When the onion is golden brown, add the pepper, and sauté, and after a few minutes add the tomatoes, salt, pepper, paprika, and cumin.
3. Cook for a few minutes and then form 8 grooves where you will then insert the eggs. Cook for 5 minutes, season with salt and pepper and then turn off.
4. Put the eggs and vegetables on the plates, sprinkle with the chopped parsley and serve.

Strawberry, Banana, and Raspberry Smoothie (Italy)

Preparation time: 15 minutes

Servings: 4

Calories for serving: 190

Macronutrients

- Carbs: 31 g
- Proteins: 8 g
- Fat: 3 g

Ingredients

- 7 oz raspberries
- 7 oz strawberries
- 14 oz bananas
- 1 glass milk

Directions

1. Wash and dry strawberries and raspberries and then cut them in half.
2. Peel the bananas and then cut them into pieces.
3. Put the strawberries, raspberries, and bananas in the blender glass and add the milk.
4. Close the blender and blend for 2 minutes.
5. Pour the smoothie into 4 glasses and serve.

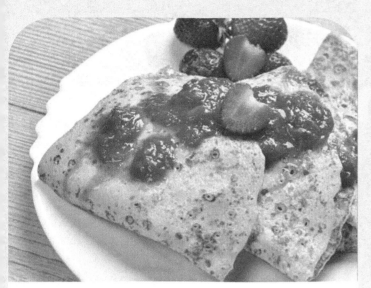

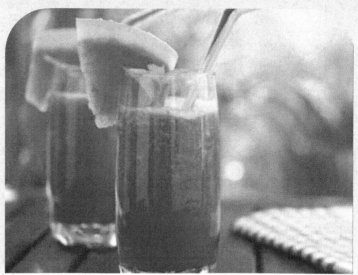

Strawberry Omelette (France)

Preparation time: 20 minutes
Cooking time: 20 minutes
Servings: 4
Calories for serving: 378

Macronutrients
- Carbs: 23 g
- Proteins: 2 g
- Fat: 8 g

Ingredients
- 4 eggs
- 10.5 oz strawberries
- 6 tbsp low-sugar strawberry jam
- 2 tbsp milk
- A pinch salt
- Mint leaves to taste

Directions

1. Wash and dry the strawberries, then cut them into cubes. Put them in a saucepan and add the jam. Cook for 10 minutes then turn off and set aside.
2. Break the eggs into a bowl and add the milk. Beat them vigorously with a fork until you get a homogeneous mixture.
3. Heat a non-stick pan and add some mixture. Cook for 2 minutes on each side, then move on to cooking the other omelets.
4. Put the omelets on 4 plates, season with the jam and strawberries, sprinkle with mint leaves, close them into two parts and serve.

Watermelon Smoothie (Italy)

Preparation time: 20 minutes + 1 hour to rest
Servings: 4
Calories for serving: 106

Macronutrients
- Carbs: 17 g
- Proteins: 2 g
- Fat: 2 g

Ingredients
- 14 oz watermelon pulp
- ½ lemon
- 2 tbsp honey

Directions

1. Wash and dry the watermelon pulp and remove the seeds.
2. Put the watermelon in a bowl and add the sugar and lemon juice. Mix well and then refrigerate to rest for 1 hour.
3. After the hour, take the watermelon from the fridge and put all the contents of the bowl in the glass of the blender.
4. Operate the blender and blend until you get a smooth and homogeneous mixture.
5. Put the smoothie in 4 glasses and serve.

Pasta, Grain, and Rice

Recipes

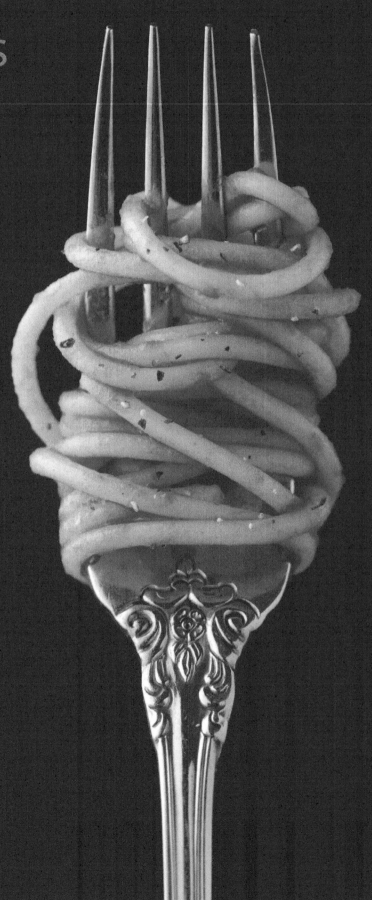

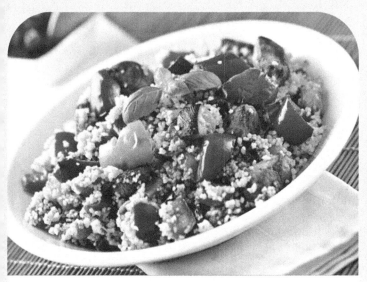

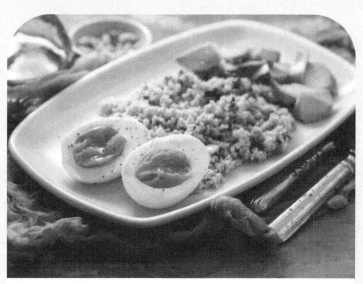

Cous Cous Salad

Preparation time: 30 minutes
Servings: 4
Calories for serving: 329

Macronutrients

- Carbs: 51 g
- Proteins: 12 g
- Fat: 10 g

Ingredients

- 11.2 oz pre-cooked couscous
- 2 cups hot vegetable broth
- 1 red pepper
- 1 yellow pepper
- 3 lemons
- Mint leaves to taste
- 1 clove garlic
- Olive oil to taste
- Salt and pepper to taste

Directions

1. Put the couscous in a bowl. Add 2 tablespoons of olive oil and salt and mix well. Pour the broth over the couscous, cover the bowl with cling film and set aside to rehydrate.

2. Meanwhile, wash the peppers, remove the seeds, and white filaments, and then cut them into cubes.

3. Put the peppers in the bowl with the couscous and add the chopped mint leaves.

4. Squeeze the lemons, slice the garlic, and transfer everything to the blender glass. Add olive oil, salt, pepper, and other mint leaves and blend until you get a thick and homogeneous sauce.

5. Pour the emulsion into the bowl with the couscous and mix well. Divide the couscous salad into plates and serve.

Cous Cous with Eggs and Tuna (Italy)

Preparation time: 20 minutes
Cooking time: 10 minutes
Servings: 4
Calories for serving: 450

Macronutrients

- Carbs: 50 g
- Proteins: 24 g
- Fat: 11 g

Ingredients

- 8.8 oz precooked couscous
- 2 zucchinis
- 5.6 oz drained canned tuna
- 4 eggs
- 1 cup hot water
- 1 lemon
- Chopped parsley to taste
- Salt and pepper to taste
- Olive oil to taste

Directions

1. Pour the couscous into a bowl and cover it with warm slightly salted water. Let it swell for 10 minutes. Then shell the couscous with a fork and season with the juice of half a lemon.

2. Meanwhile, put the eggs in a saucepan and cover them with water. Bring to a boil and continue cooking for another 8 minutes. After cooking, drain the eggs, pass them under cold water, shell them, and cut them into 8 wedges.

3. Wash and dry the zucchinis, then cut them into small cubes. Put the zucchini, tuna, and eggs in the bowl with the couscous.

4. Season with salt, pepper, oil, and the juice of the remaining half lemon. Mix well, divide into plates, and serve.

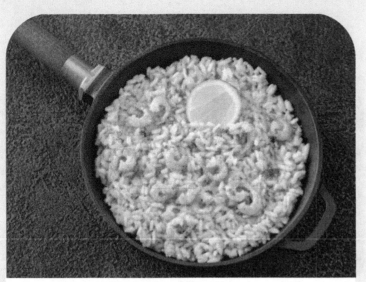

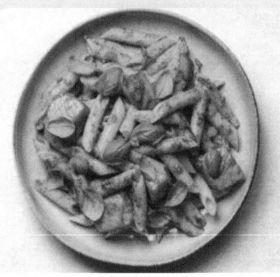

Garides Pilafi, Risotto with Shrimps (Greece)

Preparation time: 20 minutes
Cooking time: 50 minutes
Servings: 4
Calories for serving: 411

Macronutrients

- Carbs: 46 g
- Proteins: 26 g
- Fat: 9 g

Ingredients

- 35 oz shrimps
- 11.2 oz rice
- 10.5 oz tomato puree
- 1 onion
- 2 cups fish broth
- Chopped parsley to taste
- Salt and pepper to taste
- Olive oil to taste

Directions

1. Peel the onion and then chop it. Shell the shrimps, remove the intestinal filament, then wash and dry them.

2. Heat a little oil in a pan and then put the onion to brown. Then add the tomato puree. Season with salt and pepper and cook for 10 minutes.

3. After 10 minutes, add the fish broth and rice. Cook for 20 minutes, stirring often and adding more broth if necessary. After 20 minutes, add the shrimp and cook for another 15 minutes.

4. Once cooked, put the rice and shrimp on the plates, sprinkle with the chopped parsley, and serve.

Pasta with Basil and Salmon

Preparation time: 20 minutes
Cooking time: 15 minutes
Servings: 4
Calories for serving: 646

Macronutrients

- Carbs: 66 g
- Proteins: 22 g
- Fat: 14 g

Ingredients

- 9.8 oz penne
- 7 oz smoked salmon
- 1 bunch basil
- 1.7 oz flaked almonds
- 1 clove garlic
- Olive oil to taste
- Salt and pepper to taste

Directions

1. Bring a pot of water and salt to a boil and then pour in the penne. Cook for 10 minutes.

2. Meanwhile, wash and dry the basil. Transfer the basil to a glass blender and add the almonds, salt, pepper, and 4 tablespoons of olive oil.

3. Blend until you get a thick and homogeneous sauce. Put the basil sauce in a bowl.

4. Drain the pasta and put it in the bowl with the basil sauce. Add the salmon cut into small pieces and mix well.

5. Put the pasta on the plates and serve.

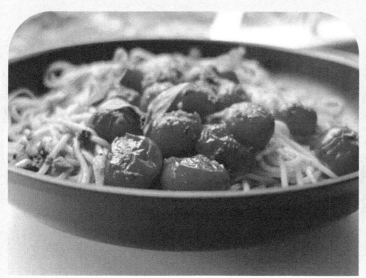

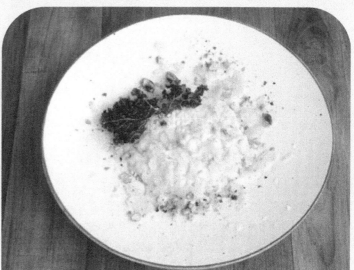

Pasta with Cherry Tomatoes and Tapenade

Preparation time: 20 minutes
Cooking time:
Servings: 4
Calories for serving: 585

Macronutrients

- Carbs: 56 g
- Proteins: 5 g
- Fat: 8 g

Ingredients

- 9.8 oz spaghetti
- 20 cherry tomatoes
- 4.2 oz black olives
- 2 tbsp capers
- 2 anchovy fillets
- 1 minced clove garlic
- Salt and pepper to taste
- Olive oil to taste

Directions

1. Chop the olives, capers, and anchovy fillets. Wash the cherry tomatoes and then cut them into 4 wedges.

2. Chop the garlic and brown it in a pan with hot olive oil. Put the cherry tomatoes and cook for 5 minutes.

3. Meanwhile, put a pot of water and salt to boil and pour the spaghetti and cook for 8 minutes.

4. After 5 minutes, add the tapenade to the tomatoes, season with salt and pepper, and mix well. Continue cooking for another 5 minutes and then turn off.

5. Drain the pasta and put it in the pan with the cherry tomatoes. Mix well, then put the spaghetti on the plates and serve.

Pilaf with Pistachios (Turkey)

Preparation time: 30 minutes
Cooking time: 30 minutes
Servings: 4
Calories for serving: 537

Macronutrients

- Carbs: 63 g
- Proteins: 8 g
- Fat: 15 g

Ingredients

- 11.2 oz basmati rice
- 3.5 oz shelled pistachios
- 2 tbsp seed oil
- 1 tsp sugar
- 2 cups boiling chicken broth
- 1 tbsp chopped parsley
- Salt and pepper to taste
- Olive oil to taste

Directions

1. Put the rice in a bowl. Add a tablespoon of salt and cover it with boiling water. Leave it immersed until the water has cooled completely. As soon as the water has cooled, drain the rice, and set it aside.

2. Put the seed oil in a saucepan and over low heat sauté the pistachios until they take on a nice golden color.

3. When the pistachios are golden brown, remove them and add olive oil and rice. Mix well, cook for a couple of minutes, and then add the pistachios, sugar, and broth.

4. Cover, season with salt and pepper, and cook for 20 minutes, stirring occasionally. After cooking, let it rest for 10 minutes, then put the rice on the plates and serve.

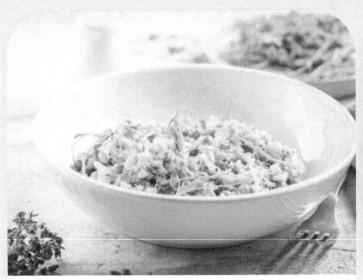

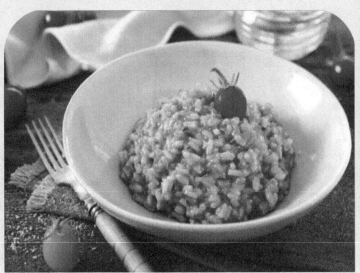

Risotto with Broccoli Cream (Italy)

Preparation time: 20 minutes
Cooking time: 40 minutes
Servings: 4
Calories for serving: 500

Macronutrients

- Carbs: 51 g
- Proteins: 5 g
- Fat: 8 g

Ingredients

- 9.8 oz rice
- 14 oz broccoli
- 3 tbsp grated Parmesan cheese
- Vegetable broth to taste
- Salt and pepper to taste
- Olive oil to taste

Directions

1. Divide the broccoli into tops, wash them and then cook them for 10 minutes in boiling salted water. Put the broccoli and a little cooking water in a bowl and blend them with an immersion blender.

2. Put some oil in a saucepan and let it heat up. Put the rice and toast it for 2 minutes. Now add some vegetable broth and stir until completely absorbed. Continue in the same way until the rice is cooked.

3. Once cooked, add the broccoli cream and Parmesan cheese, and continue cooking for another 5 minutes, always continuing to mix.

4. Season with salt and pepper and turn off. Divide the risotto into plates and serve.

Risotto with Tomato (Italy)

Preparation time: 15 minutes
Cooking time: 40 minutes
Servings: 4
Calories for serving: 550

Macronutrients

- Carbs: 62 g
- Proteins: 13 g
- Fat: 12 g

Ingredients

- 8.4 oz rice
- 17.6 oz peeled tomatoes
- 8 basil leaves
- ½ onion
- 4 cup vegetable broth
- 1.7 oz grated Parmesan cheese
- 1 pinch sugar
- Olive oil to taste
- Salt and pepper to taste

Directions

1. Peel the onion and then chop it. Heat a little oil in a pan and then put the onion to brown. Add the chopped basil and the peeled tomato. Mix well, then season with salt and pepper, add a pinch of sugar and cook for 20 minutes.

2. Put a drizzle of oil in a saucepan and, as soon as it is hot, put the rice to toast for 2 minutes. Add the tomato sauce, mix well and as soon as it is absorbed, start adding a little broth at a time. Stir constantly and as soon as the broth has been absorbed, add the other. Continue in the same way until cooked.

3. When the rice is cooked, add the Parmesan, and stir until completely incorporated. Then put the risotto on the plates and serve.

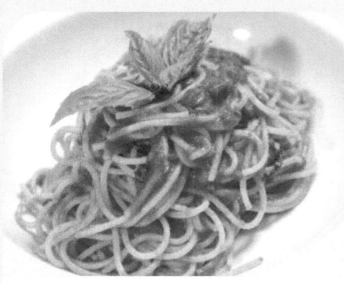

Spaghetti Alla Marinara

Preparation time: 15 minutes
Cooking time: 15 minutes
Servings: 4
Calories for serving: 565

Macronutrients

- Carbs: 56 g
- Proteins: 7 g
- Fat: 8 g

Ingredients

- 9.8 oz spaghetti
- 17.6 oz peeled tomatoes
- 2 cloves garlic
- Dried oregano to taste
- Olive oil to taste
- Salt and pepper to taste

Directions

1. Peel the garlic cloves and then cut them into thin slices. Put a little oil in a pan and put the wedges to brown for 2 minutes.

2. Now pour the peeled tomatoes and mash them with a wooden spoon. Season with salt and pepper and cook for 5 minutes.

3. In the meantime, put a pot of water and salt to boil and, when it starts to boil, pour in the spaghetti. Cook for 8–10 minutes, then drain the pasta and put it in the pan with the tomatoes.

4. Mix well, add the oregano, and cook for another 2 minutes.

5. After cooking, put the pasta on the plates and serve.

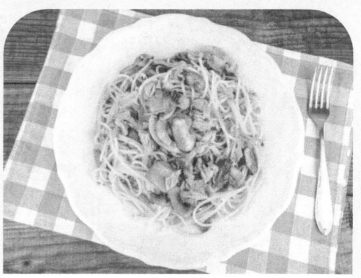

Spaghetti with Tuna and Mushrooms (Italy)

Preparation time: 20 minutes
Cooking time: 30 minutes
Servings: 4
Calories for serving: 659

Macronutrients

- Carbs: 65 g
- Proteins: 21 g
- Fat: 9 g

Ingredients

- 9.8 oz spaghetti
- 1 onion
- 1 clove garlic
- 7 oz champignon mushrooms
- 7 oz drained tuna in oil
- ½ glass white wine
- Chopped parsley to taste
- Salt and pepper to taste

Directions

1. Peel the onion and garlic and then chop them. Wash the mushrooms, dry them, and then cut them into slices.

2. Put a little oil in a pan and, when it is hot, put the onion and garlic to brown. Add the mushrooms and deglaze with the white wine. When the wine has evaporated, add the tuna, salt, pepper, and parsley, and cook for 10 minutes.

3. Meanwhile, bring a pot of water and salt to a boil and pour the spaghetti. Cook for 8–10 minutes, then drain the pasta and put it in the pan with the mushrooms.

4. Mix well, cook for 2 minutes, and then turn off. Put the pasta and the sauce on the plates and serve.

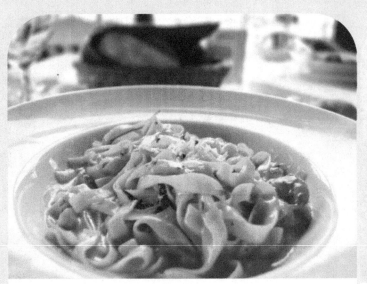

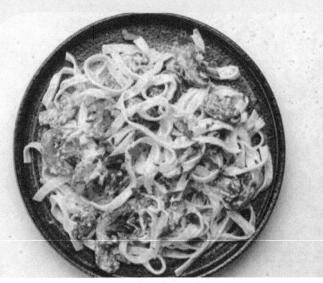

Tagliatelle with Pepper Cream (Italy)

Preparation time: 20 minutes
Cooking time: 25 minutes
Servings: 4
Calories for serving: 565

Macronutrients

- Carbs: 63 g
- Proteins: 13 g
- Fat: 10 g

Ingredients

- 9.8 oz tagliatelle
- 3 red peppers
- 1 onion
- 1 clove garlic
- 4 tbsp grated Parmesan cheese
- 8 basil leaves
- Salt and pepper to taste
- Olive oil to taste

Directions

1. Wash the peppers, cut them into slices, and remove seeds and white filaments. Peel the onion and cut it into slices. Peel and chop the garlic clove.

2. Heat a little oil in a pan and then put the garlic to brown. Now add the onion and peppers and mix. Then add the chopped basil, season with salt and pepper, and cook for 20 minutes.

3. Meanwhile, bring a pot of water and salt to a boil and cook tagliatelle for10 minutes, or until indicated on the package.

4. Once the peppers are cooked, transfer them together with all the contents of the pan into the glass blender and blend until you get a nice red cream.

5. Put the cream in a bowl. When the pasta is cooked, drain it, and put it in the bowl with the pepper cream. Mix well, then add the Parmesan and mix again. Now put the pasta on the plates and serve.

Tagliatelle with Porcini Mushrooms

Preparation time: 25 minutes
Cooking time: 20 minutes
Servings: 4
Calories for serving: 506

Macronutrients

- Carbs: 63 g
- Proteins: 10 g
- Fat: 12 g

Ingredients

- 10.5 oz porcini mushrooms
- 9.8 oz tagliatelle
- 1 clove minced garlic
- Chopped parsley to taste
- 1 minced hot red pepper
- 1 glass vegetable broth
- Salt and pepper to taste
- Olive oil to taste

Directions

1. Wash the mushrooms with a damp cloth and then cut them into small pieces.

2. Heat a round of oil in a pan and add the garlic and parsley. Fry for 2 minutes and then add the mushrooms. Add the hot red pepper, stir, and cook for 5 minutes.

3. After 5 minutes, season with salt and pepper, add the broth and cook for another 10 minutes.

4. Meanwhile, bring a pot of water and salt to a boil, add the tagliatelle, and cook for 8 minutes. Once cooked, drain the tagliatelle, and place them in the pan with the mushrooms.

5. Mix well, cook for 2 minutes, and then turn off. Put the pasta on the plates and serve.

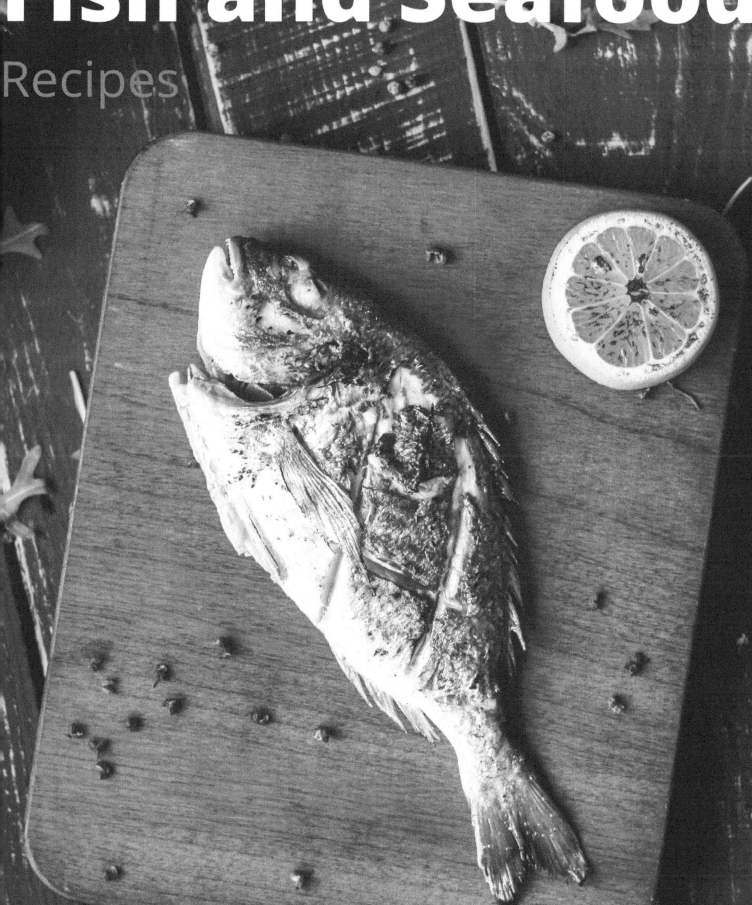

Fish and Seafood

Recipes

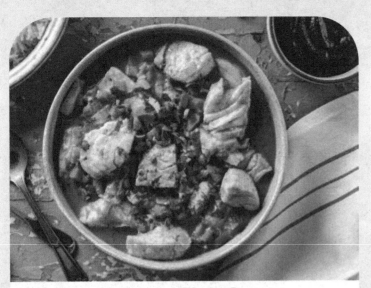

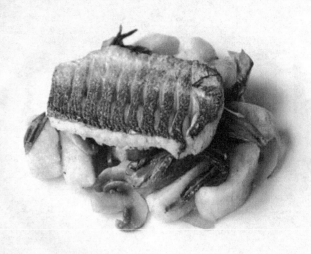

Aljotta: Maltese Fish Soup (Malta)

Preparation time: 30 minutes
Cooking time: 30 minutes
Servings: 4
Calories for serving: 245

Macronutrients

- Carbs: 3 g
- Proteins: 21 g
- Fat: 12 g

Ingredients

- 35 oz mixed fish for soup
- 17.5 oz tomatoes
- 1 chopped onion
- 1 tbsp chopped carrot
- 1 tbsp chopped celery
- 1 clove minced garlic
- 4 mint leaves
- 1 sprig marjoram
- Salt and pepper to taste
- Olive oil to taste

Directions

1. Clean the fish from scales, bones, and entrails. Remove the heads and then wash them. Put them in a pot with 4 cups of water, the onion, and celery, and cook for 15 minutes.

2. Meanwhile, heat a little oil in a pan and fry the garlic. Add the diced tomatoes, mint leaves, and marjoram and cook for 2 minutes.

3. Now add the filtered fish broth and let it boil for 5 minutes so that the sauce thickens a little.

4. Now cut the fish into cubes and put it in the pan. Continue cooking for another 10 minutes. Season with salt and pepper, mix well and then turn off.

5. Put the soup on the plates, season with a little oil, and serve.

Baked Sea Bream with Porcini Mushrooms (Italy)

Preparation time: 25 minutes
Cooking time: 30 minutes
Servings: 4
Calories for serving: 382

Macronutrients

- Carbs: 20 g
- Proteins: 40 g
- Fat: 6 g

Ingredients

- 4 sea bream fillets of 7 oz each
- 4 porcini mushrooms
- 4 medium potatoes
- 2 sprigs rosemary
- 1 clove minced garlic
- Salt and pepper to taste
- Olive oil to taste

Directions

1. Peel the potatoes, wash them, and then cut them into thin slices. Remove the earthy part of the mushrooms, wash them, and then cut them into slices. Brush a baking pan with olive oil and put the mushrooms and potatoes inside. Season with oil, salt, and pepper and put in the oven. Cook at 392°F for 10 minutes.

2. Meanwhile, wash the sea bream fillets, pat them with a paper towel and remove all the bones.

3. After 10 minutes, take the baking pan from the oven and put the sea bream inside. Season with salt and pepper and sprinkle with minced garlic. Add the rosemary and return the baking pan to the oven.

4. Continue cooking for 20 minutes and at 356°F. After cooking, remove the baking pan from the oven and let it rest for a couple of minutes.

5. Then put the sea bream fillets on the plates, add the potatoes and mushrooms, and serve.

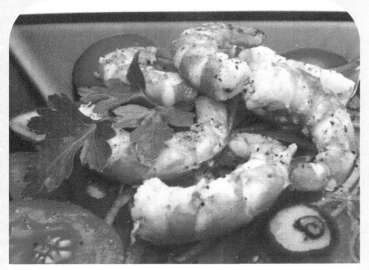

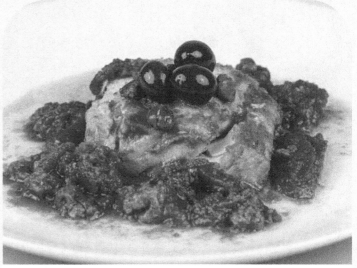

Catalan-Style Shrimps (Spain)

Preparation time: 25 minutes
Cooking time: 5 minutes
Servings: 4
Calories for serving: 268

Macronutrients

- Carbs: 6 g
- Proteins: 20 g
- Fat: 8 g

Ingredients

- 21.1 oz shrimps
- 7 oz ripe red tomatoes
- 7 oz white onion
- 4 chopped basil leaves
- White wine vinegar to taste
- Salt and pepper to taste
- Olive oil to taste

Directions

1. Wash the tomatoes, cut them into cubes, and put them in a bowl. Add oil, salt, pepper, and basil leaves, mix well, and set aside.

2. Peel the onion and cut it into slices. Put the onion in a bowl and add the vinegar. Cover the onion with cold water and set aside.

3. Shell the shrimps, remove the intestinal filament, wash, and dry them. Heat a little oil in a pan and, when it is hot, put the prawns to cook. Cook for 3–4 minutes, season with salt and pepper and turn off.

4. Now take the onion, drain it, and put it in the bowl with the tomatoes. Add the shrimp seasoned with a drizzle of oil, then divide into serving plates and serve.

Cod with Onions (Italy)

Preparation time: 20 minutes
Cooking time: 30 minutes
Servings: 4
Calories for serving: 227

Macronutrients

- Carbs: 10 g
- Proteins: 29 g
- Fat: 9 g

Ingredients

- 28.2 oz cod fillet
- 17.6 oz peeled tomato
- 9 onions
- ½ glass white wine
- 3.5 oz black olives
- Flour to taste
- Salt and pepper to taste
- Olive oil to taste

Directions

1. Wash and dry the cod, remove the bones and skin, and then cut it into slices. Put the flour on a plate and flour the cod on both sides.

2. Heat some oil in a pan and, when it is hot enough, put the cod to cook. Cook for 5 minutes on each side, then turn off and set aside.

3. Meanwhile, peel the onions, cut them into slices and put them to stew in a pan with hot oil for 5 minutes. Add a little water and cook for 5 minutes. Then add the white wine and let it evaporate. Then add the tomato, season with salt and pepper, and cook for another 10 minutes.

4. Now put the cod and black olives in the pan with the onions and cook for another 10 minutes.

5. When cooked, turn off, put the cod, olives, and onions on the plates, sprinkle with the cooking juices, and serve.

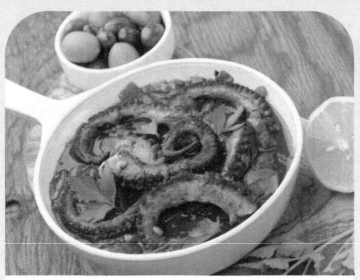

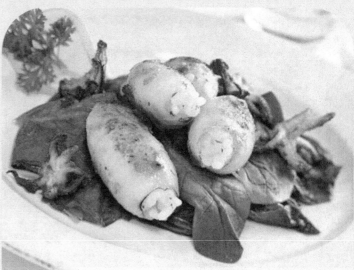

Crasato Chtapodi, Octopus in Wine (Greece)

Preparation time: 20 minutes
Cooking time: 40 minutes
Servings: 4
Calories for serving: 282

Macronutrients

- Carbs: 4 g
- Proteins: 28 g
- Fat: 10 g

Ingredients

- 28.2 oz pre-cleaned octopus
- 2 cups red wine
- 16 cherry tomatoes
- 1 bay leaf
- 2 sage leaves
- Salt and pepper to taste
- Olive oil to taste

Directions

1. Wash the octopus and then cut it into small pieces. Put it in a saucepan together with 4 tablespoons of olive oil and let it cook until its water has completely evaporated. At this point, season with salt and pepper.

2. Now add the wine and cook for 25 minutes, or until the octopus is soft and the cooking juices thick.

3. Now wash the cherry tomatoes, then cut them in half and put them in the saucepan, together with the bay leaf and sage.

4. Cook for another 10 minutes, then turn off and remove the sage and bay leaves. Put the octopus and cherry tomatoes on the plate, sprinkle with the cooking juices and serve.

Kalamarakia Yemista, Greek Stuffed Calamari (Greece)

Preparation time: 25 minutes
Cooking time: 65 minutes
Servings: 4
Calories for serving: 455

Macronutrients

- Carbs: 25 g
- Proteins: 37 g
- Fat: 8 g

Ingredients

- 28.2 oz pre-cleaned calamari
- 1 cup rice
- 1 cup spring onions
- 4 sprigs dill
- Salt and pepper to taste
- Olive oil to taste

Directions

1. Wash and dry the calamari well. Then cut the tentacles into small pieces.

2. Wash the onions, cut them into thin slices, and put them to stew in a pan with hot olive oil. Cook for 3 minutes and then add the tentacles.

3. When the cooking water of the tentacles has evaporated, add 3 tablespoons of olive oil. Stir with a spatula and add the rice, stirring constantly.

4. Now add ½ cup water and the dill and let it boil briefly until the water has completely evaporated leaving only the oil as a cooking liquid.

5. Now take the calamari and fill them with rice, leaving some space on the bottom. Close the bottom of the calamari with toothpicks and place them in a saucepan. Add 4 tablespoons of oil and cover them with cold water. Let them boil slowly for 45 minutes, allowing all the water to evaporate completely.

6. Once cooked, put the squid and the cooking juices on the plates and serve.

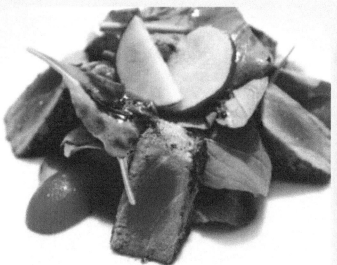

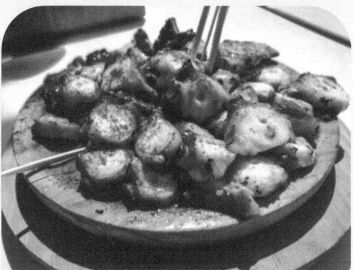

Marinated Tuna with Tomatoes (Italy)

Preparation time: 20 minutes + 3 hours of marinating
Cooking time: 15 minutes
Servings: 4
Calories for serving: 282

Macronutrients

- Carbs: 5 g
- Proteins: 38 g
- Fat: 6 g

Ingredients

- 4 steaks of tuna of 5.2 oz each
- 1 clove minced garlic
- 1 tbsp fennel seeds
- ½ glass white wine
- 1 lemon
- 2 tomatoes
- 2 tbsp chopped rosemary
- Chopped parsley to taste
- Salt and pepper to taste
- Olive oil to taste

Directions

1. Put the fennel seeds, rosemary, salt, pepper, and wine in a bowl. Mix well and then put the tuna slices. Put them in the fridge and let them marinate for 3 hours.

2. After 3 hours, take the tuna out of the fridge. Brush a baking pan with olive oil and put the tuna inside. Wash the tomatoes, cut them into cubes, and put them in the baking pan with the tuna.

3. Sprinkle with the marinade and chopped garlic. Wash the lemons, cut them into rings, and place them on top of the tuna. Place the baking pan in the oven and bake at 356°F for 15 minutes.

4. Once cooked, take the baking pan out of the oven, put the tuna, lemon slices and tomatoes on serving plates, sprinkle with the cooking juices, chopped parsley and serve.

Octopus with Paprika (Spain)

Preparation time: 30 minutes
Cooking time: 55 minutes
Servings: 4
Calories for serving: 268

Macronutrients

- Carbs: 7 g
- Proteins: 32 g
- Fat: 10 g

Ingredients

- 35 oz pre-cleaned octopus
- Spicy paprika to taste
- 1 carrot
- 1 onion
- 2 bay leaves
- Salt to taste
- Olive oil to taste

Directions

1. Wash and dry the octopus. Peel the carrot and onion and then cut them into not too small pieces. Wash the bay leaves.

2. Put carrot, onion, salt, and bay leaf in a pot full of water and bring to a boil. Then put the octopus inside and cook for 45 minutes. After cooking, turn it off and let the octopus cool in the pot.

3. Heat a grill and, when it is hot, put the drained octopus to cook. Grill for 10 minutes, mashing it with a fork, then place it on a cutting board and cut it into small pieces.

4. Put the octopus pieces in a bowl. Season them with oil, salt and paprika. Mix well, then divide the octopus into plates and serve.

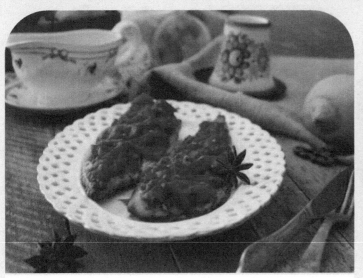

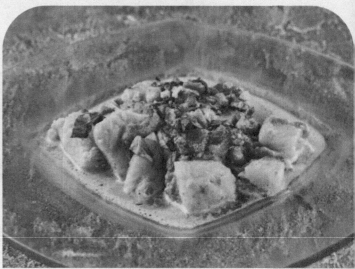

Plakì, Greek Mackerel (Greece)

Preparation time: 25 minutes
Cooking time: 25 minutes
Servings: 4
Calories for serving: 207

Macronutrients

- Carbs: 4 g
- Proteins: 32 g
- Fat: 10 g

Ingredients

- 4 mackerel fillets of 7 oz each
- 2 minced garlic cloves
- 2 ripe red tomatoes
- Chopped parsley to taste
- Salt and pepper to taste
- Olive oil to taste

Directions

1. Wash the mackerel fillets and remove all the bones present.

2. Brush a baking pan with olive oil and put the mackerel fillets inside. Season the fish with salt and pepper.

3. Wash the tomatoes, peel them, cut them into cubes, and place them on top of the fish. Sprinkle with the garlic and chopped parsley as well.

4. Add ½ glass of olive oil and a cup of water and put the baking pan in the oven. Cook at 392°F for 15 minutes and at 356°F for 10 minutes. After cooking, pre-wash the baking pan from the oven and let it rest for a few minutes. Then put the fish and tomatoes on the plates and serve.

Provençal Sea Bream (France)

Preparation time: 25 minutes
Cooking time: 40 minutes
Servings: 4
Calories for serving: 246

Macronutrients

- Carbs: 7 g
- Proteins: 35 g
- Fat: 10 g

Ingredients

- 4 sea bream fillets of 7 oz each
- 1 fennel
- 2 green peppers
- 1 onion
- 3.5 oz cherry tomatoes
- Salt and pepper to taste
- Olive oil to taste

Directions

1. Wash and dry the sea bream fillets and remove all the bones present.

2. Clean the fennel well, removing the beard and the hardest leaves, then wash it and cut it into cubes. Wash the peppers, remove the seeds, and cut them into cubes. Wash the tomatoes and then divide them in half. Peel and then chop the onion.

3. Heat some oil in a pan and then add the fennel. Cook for 10 minutes, then season with salt and pepper and turn off.

4. Brush a baking pan with olive oil and add the tomatoes, peppers, chopped onion, and stewed fennel. Season with salt and pepper and then put the sea bream fillets on top. Season the fish with salt and pepper, add a drizzle of oil, and put the baking pan in the oven. Cook at 356°F for 30 minutes.

5. After cooking, take the sea bream from the oven. Then put the sea bream fillets on serving plates, add the vegetables and serve.

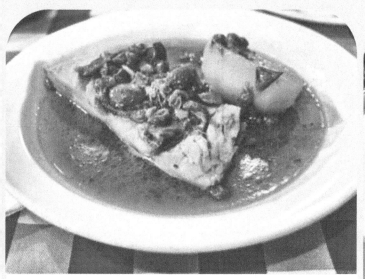

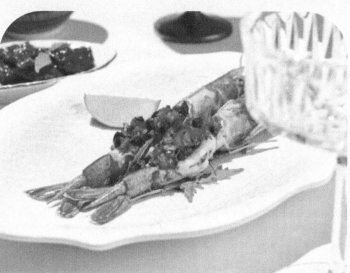

Psarosoupa - Greek Fish Soup

Preparation time: 25 minutes
Cooking time: 40 minutes
Servings: 4
Calories for serving: 375

Macronutrients

- Carbs: 22 g
- Proteins: 30 g
- Fat: 8 g

Ingredients

- 28.2 oz cod fillet
- 4 potatoes
- 4 spring onions
- 2 carrots
- 2 stalks of celery
- 2 tomatoes
- 2 eggs
- 1 lemon
- 1 cup rice
- Salt and pepper to taste
- Olive oil to taste

Directions

1. Remove the cod skin and bones, wash it, and pat it dry with a paper towel. Season the fish with salt and pepper and set aside.

2. Peel the potatoes, carrots, and onions, peel the celery, and then wash all the vegetables. Put the whole vegetables in a saucepan covered with water and bring them to a boil.

3. Wash the tomatoes, cut them into cubes, and when the water starts to boil, put them in the saucepan with the other vegetables. Cook for 10 minutes, then add the fish, salt and pepper, and more water if necessary.

4. Cook for another 20 minutes, then remove the cod and vegetables from the saucepan and place them in a bowl. Filter the broth and put it back in the saucepan. Blend the fish and vegetables with the hand blender.

5. Put the broth back on the heat and, as soon as it starts to boil, pour in the rice and the fish and vegetable smoothie.

   Meanwhile, prepare the sauce. Beat the eggs well in a bowl and slowly add the lemon juice. Take some broth with a ladle and pour it slowly into the sauce, whisking constantly.

Scampi Alla Busara (Montenegro)

Preparation time: 25 minutes
Cooking time: 25 minutes
Servings: 4
Calories for serving: 168

Macronutrients

- Carbs: 11 g
- Proteins: 19 g
- Fat: 5 g

Ingredients

- 35 oz scampi
- ½ glass white wine
- 1 clove minced garlic
- 1 fresh chili, chopped
- 10.5 oz peeled tomatoes
- 2 tbsp chopped parsley
- Salt and pepper to taste
- Olive oil to taste

Directions

1. With a sharp knife make a vertical cut on the back of the scampi and remove the intestinal filament. Then wash them and let them drain.

2. Heat a little oil in a pan and then brown the garlic. Then add the chili and scampi.

3. Add the white wine and let it evaporate. Then add the peeled tomatoes and season with salt and pepper.

4. Cover the pan with a lid and cook for 15 minutes.

5. After cooking, put the scampi and the cooking juices on the plates. Sprinkle with chopped parsley and serve.

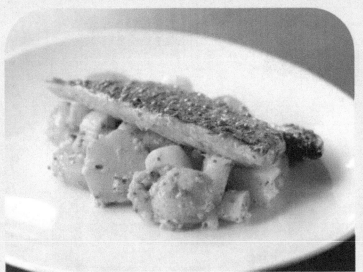

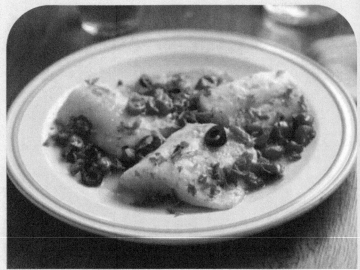

Sea Bass and Potatoes in Sauce (Spain)

Preparation time: 25 minutes
Cooking time: 40 minutes
Servings: 4
Calories for serving: 398

Macronutrients

- Carbs: 25 g
- Proteins: 40 g
- Fat: 9 g

Ingredients

- 4 sea bass fillets of 8.8 oz each
- 17.6 oz potatoes
- 2 minced garlic cloves
- 2 minced spicy red pepper
- 3 tbsp powdered pink pepper
- 2 cups water
- 1 tbsp flour
- Salt to taste
- Olive oil to taste

Directions

1. Wash and dry the sea bass and remove all the bones and skin. Peel the potatoes, wash them, and cut them into thin slices.

2. Heat a few tablespoons of olive oil in a pan and add the garlic and red pepper. Sauté for a couple of minutes and then add the flour and pink pepper. Toast for a few seconds and then add the water.

3. Mix well and then add the potatoes. Cook for 20 minutes, stirring occasionally. After 20 minutes, add the fish and cook for another 15 minutes.

4. After 15 minutes, season with salt and then turn off. Put the sea bass and potatoes on the plates, sprinkle with the sauce, and serve.

Stewed Cod with Olives (Italy)

Preparation time: 20 minutes
Cooking time: 25 minutes
Servings: 4
Calories for serving: 329

Macronutrients

- Carbs: 4 g
- Proteins: 42 g
- Fat: 7 g

Ingredients

- 28.2 oz cod fillet
- 2 minced garlic cloves
- 1.7 oz black olives
- 4 tomatoes
- 1 tbsp capers
- 1 onion
- Dried oregano to taste
- Olive oil to taste

Directions

1. Remove the skin and bones from the cod, then wash and dry it. Cut the cod into slices. Peel the onion and then cut it into thin slices.

2. Heat a little oil in a saucepan and then put the garlic and onion to sauté. Cook for a couple of minutes and then add the cod. Cook for 1 minute on each side, then add the olives and capers, and sprinkle with oregano.

3. Add a couple of tablespoons of water and cook for 10 minutes. Then add the diced tomatoes, season with salt and pepper, and cook for another 10 minutes.

4. After cooking, turn off, and put the cod, tomatoes, olives, and capers on the plates. Sprinkle with the cooking juices and serve.

Poultry

Recipes

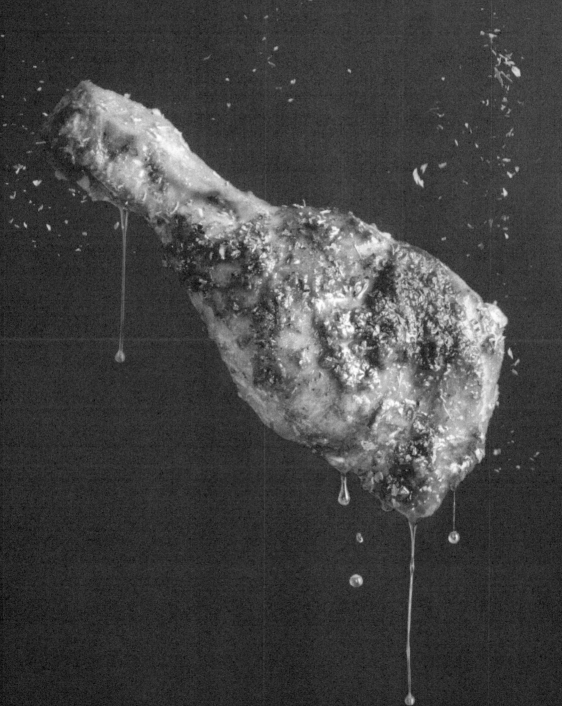

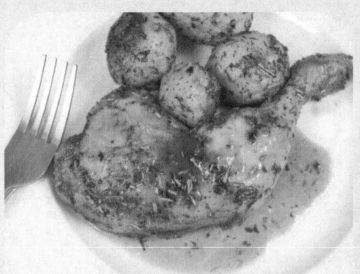
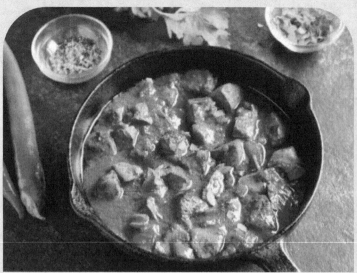

Chermoula Chicken Legs (Morocco)

Preparation time: 25 minutes
Cooking time: 45 minutes
Servings: 4
Calories for serving: 506

Macronutrients

- Carbs: 34 g
- Proteins: 46 g
- Fat: 12 g

Ingredients

- 12 chicken legs
- 28.2 oz potatoes
- 1 bunch chopped parsley
- 1 bunch chopped fresh cilantro
- 5 minced garlic cloves
- 1 tbsp cumin powder
- 1 tsp strong paprika
- 2 lemons
- Olive oil to taste
- Salt and pepper to taste

Directions

1. Start by preparing the chermoula. Put the garlic, coriander, parsley, paprika, salt and pepper, the juice of the two lemons, and 4 tablespoons of olive oil in a bowl. Stir until you get a thick and homogeneous sauce.

2. Remove the skin from the chicken legs. Put them in a bowl and cover them with the chermoula. Peel the potatoes, wash them, and then cut them into cubes. Put them in the bowl with the chicken and mix well.

3. Brush a baking pan with olive oil and then pour the chicken and potatoes inside. Season with salt and pepper and put the baking pan in the oven. Cook at 392°F for 45 minutes.

4. Once cooked, take the baking pan out of the oven, put the chicken and potatoes on the plates, and serve.

Chicken and Turkey Stew (Italy)

Preparation time: 20 minutes
Cooking time: 25 minutes
Servings: 4
Calories for serving: 336

Macronutrients

- Carbs: 8 g
- Proteins: 44 g
- Fat: 7 g

Ingredients

- 14 oz chicken breast
- 14 oz turkey breast
- 1 clove garlic
- 2 cups vegetable broth
- Flour to taste
- 2 tbsp tomato sauce
- 1 sprig rosemary
- 1 sprig thyme
- 4 juniper berries
- Salt and pepper to taste
- Olive oil to taste

Directions

1. Remove the excess fat from the chicken and turkey and then cut the meat into cubes. Put the meat in a bowl and add salt, pepper, and flour. Stir until the meat is well-floured.

2. Peel the garlic clove and then chop it. Wash and dry the thyme and rosemary and then chop them.

3. Heat 2 tablespoons of olive oil in a pan. When the oil is hot, add the garlic and herbs and sauté for 2 minutes. Then add the chicken and turkey and sauté for 3 minutes.

4. Now add the tomato puree, and broth, season with salt and pepper, and cook for 15 minutes, stirring occasionally.

5. When cooked, turn off, put the stew on serving plates and serve.

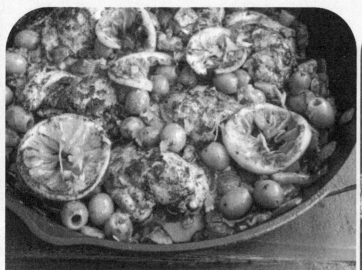 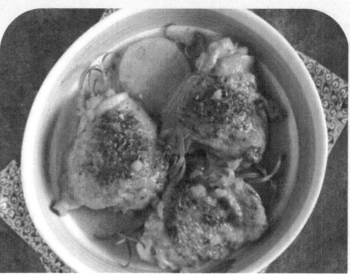

Chicken M'qalli with Olives and Lemon (Morocco)

Preparation time: 15 minutes + 2 hours of marinating
Cooking time: 80 minutes
Servings: 4
Calories for serving: 484

Macronutrients

- Carbs: 7 g
- Proteins: 35 g
- Fat: 12 g

Ingredients

- 2 chicken breasts of 14 oz each
- 3 sliced onions
- 2 minced garlic cloves
- 1 tsp saffron
- 1 tbsp lemon juice
- 1 glass water
- 10 green olives
- 2 lemons cut into slices
- Salt and pepper to taste
- Olive oil to taste

Directions

1. Put the chicken in a bowl, add salt and pepper, and let it rest for 2 hours.

2. After 2 hours, put the chicken in the tagine along with onions, garlic, saffron, ginger, lemon juice, salt, and water.

3. Cover and cook for 75 minutes.

4. Finally, add the lemon slices and olives and continue cooking for another 5 minutes over low heat.

5. Once cooked, cut the chicken into pieces, and put it on plates. Add the olives and lemon slices, sprinkle with the cooking juices and serve.

Chicken Stew with Lemon (Italy)

Preparation time: 20 minutes
Cooking time: 50 minutes
Servings: 4
Calories for serving: 327

Macronutrients

- Carbs: 8 g
- Proteins: 42 g
- Fat: 10 g

Ingredients

- 35 oz chicken cut into pieces
- 12 shallots
- 1 cup beef broth
- 2 lemons
- 1 glass white wine
- 1 stalk chopped celery
- Chopped parsley to taste
- Salt and pepper to taste
- Olive oil to taste

Directions

1. Wash the chicken pieces under running water and then pat them dry with a paper towel. Heat a drizzle of oil in a pan and brown the chicken for 4 minutes on all sides. Turn off and set aside.

2. Peel the shallots and then cut them into slices. Brush a baking pan with olive oil and put the chicken with the cooking juices and shallots inside. Season with salt and pepper and put the baking pan in the oven. Cook at 392°F for 10 minutes.

3. After 10 minutes, remove the meat from the oven and transfer everything to a saucepan. Add the celery and cook for 3 minutes. Add the white wine and let it evaporate.

4. Wash the lemons, remove the zest, cut the pulp into cubes, and put it in the saucepan with the chicken. Add the meat broth and continue cooking for another 30 minutes. When cooked, turn off, sprinkle with chopped parsley, and mix well.

5. Put the chicken on the plates, season with the cooking juices, and serve.

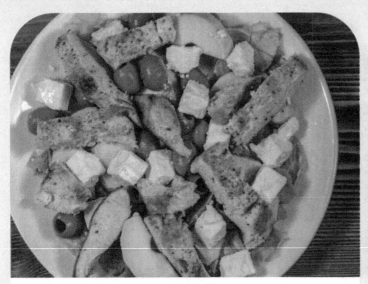 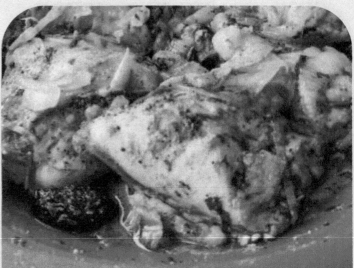

Chicken Tapas (Spain)

Preparation time: 20 minutes
Cooking time: 75 minutes
Servings: 4
Calories for serving: 342

Macronutrients

- Carbs: 5 g
- Proteins: 36 g
- Fat: 7 g

Ingredients

- 21 oz chicken breast
- 1 chicken leg
- 1 chopped red pepper
- 2 glasses of white wine
- Flour to taste
- 3.5 oz green olives
- 2 cloves minced garlic
- 1 sprig thyme
- Salt and pepper to taste
- Olive oil to taste

Directions

1. Boil the chicken leg for 40 minutes with 2 cups of water. After cooking, turn off and filter the broth. Remove the excess fat from the chicken, cut it into cubes, and put it in a bowl. Add the flour, mix, and flour the chicken well.

2. Heat 2 tablespoons of olive oil in a pan. When the oil is hot, add the chicken and brown it for 5 minutes. After 5 minutes, season with salt and pepper, drain the chicken and set aside.

3. Put the broth in the pan where you cooked the chicken and add the wine, garlic, red pepper, and thyme. Cook for 20 minutes, over medium heat, and stirring often.

4. Now add the chicken and the olives and continue cooking for another 15 minutes. Once cooked, remove the thyme, put the chicken on the plates, sprinkle with the cooking juices, and serve.

Chicken Tajine, Red Onions, and Saffron (Morocco)

Preparation time: 20 minutes
Cooking time: 50 minutes
Servings: 4
Calories for serving: 427

Macronutrients

- Carbs: 12 g
- Proteins: 40 g
- Fat: 11 g

Ingredients

- 17.6 oz apples
- 35 oz walnut kernels
- 42.3 oz chicken cut into pieces
- 6 red onions
- Cinnamon powder to taste
- 2 tbsp honey
- 3 cup chicken broth
- 2 tsp saffron
- Salt and pepper to taste
- Olive oil to taste

Directions

1. Heat 2 tablespoons of oil in a saucepan, add the chopped chicken, a sprinkle of pepper, a little cinnamon, and saffron, and brown for 5 minutes over medium heat, stirring constantly.

2. Peel the onions, cut them into pieces, and place them in the pan with the chicken. Add the broth and cook for 30 minutes.

3. Meanwhile, peel the apples, remove the seeds, and cut them into cubes. After 30 minutes, put the apples in the pan and cook for another 15 minutes.

4. Heat a non-stick pan and roast the walnuts for a minute. Then add the honey, stir, cook for 2 minutes, and then turn it off. Put the walnuts in the pan with the chicken, season with salt and pepper and cook for 2 minutes.

5. When cooked, turn off, put the chicken on the plates, add the onions, apples, and walnuts, sprinkle with the cooking juices, and serve.

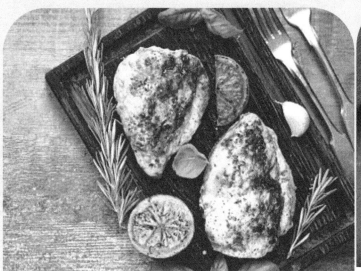
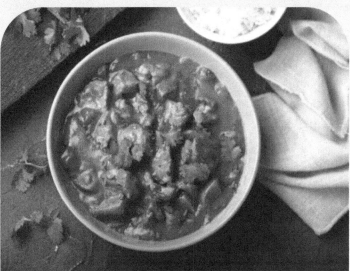

Chicken with Basil (Italy)

Preparation time: 20 minutes
Cooking time: 55 minutes
Servings: 4
Calories for serving: 335

Macronutrients

- Carbs: 9 g
- Proteins: 42 g
- Fat: 8 g

Ingredients

- 35 oz chicken cut into pieces
- 1 onion
- ½ glass white wine
- 10.5 oz peeled tomato
- 2 minced garlic cloves
- 1 tsp chopped thyme
- 2 bay leaves
- 12 basil leaves
- Salt and pepper to taste
- Olive oil to taste

Directions

1. Wash and dry the chicken. Peel the onion and then cut it into rings. Heat some olive oil in a pan and then add the onion. Cook for 3 minutes then add the chicken and garlic. Cook for 2 minutes then add thyme and bay leaves.

2. Mix well and then blend with the wine and let it evaporate. Lower the heat to low, add the tomato, season with salt and pepper, and cook for 50 minutes, turning the chicken from time to time.

3. 10 minutes before the end of cooking, chop the basil and put it in the pan with the chicken. Mix well and finish cooking.

4. Once cooked, turn off, put the chicken on the plates, season with the cooking juices, and serve.

Coriander Chicken (Algeria)

Preparation time: 20 minutes
Cooking time: 40 minutes
Servings: 4
Calories for serving: 330

Macronutrients

- Carbs: 5 g
- Proteins: 44 g
- Fat: 9 g

Ingredients

- 28.2 oz diced chicken breast
- 3.5 oz black olives
- 1 tsp turmeric powder
- 4 minced garlic cloves
- 2 tsp chopped coriander
- 1 lemon cut into slices
- Salt and pepper to taste
- Olive oil to taste

Directions

1. Heat 3 tablespoons of oil in a pan and then add the chicken.

2. When the chicken is well browned, add the garlic cloves, the spices, and the finely chopped coriander, and season with salt and pepper.

3. Cook for 10 minutes, occasionally turning the chicken pieces.

4. After 10 minutes, add as much water as you need to cover the chicken and simmer over low heat until cooked. Add more water if necessary.

5. Finally, add the olives and lemon; continue cooking for another 10 minutes over low heat or until the sauce has reduced. At this point turn off, put the chicken and the cooking juices on the serving plates and serve.

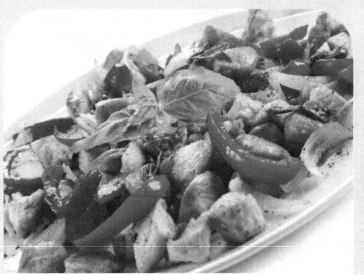

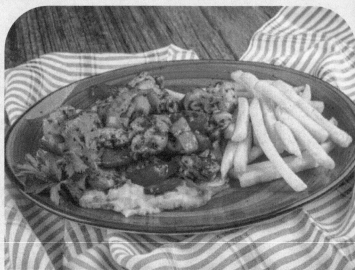

Spanish-Style Turkey (Spain)

Preparation time: 25 minutes
Cooking time: 60 minutes
Servings: 4
Calories for serving: 339

Macronutrients

- Carbs: 10 g
- Proteins: 39 g
- Fat: 9 g

Ingredients

- 21 oz turkey breast
- 1 yellow pepper
- 1 red pepper
- ½ glass white wine
- Chopped parsley to taste
- Olive oil to taste
- Salt and pepper to taste

Directions

1. Divide the peppers in two, remove the seeds and internal filaments, wash them, dry them, and cut the pulp into small pieces.

2. Cut the turkey breast into cubes and put it in a bowl. Add salt, pepper, oil, and wine and marinate for 30 minutes.

3. After 30 minutes, peel and chop the onion and brown it in a pan with hot olive oil. Add the turkey cubes and brown them for a couple of minutes, mixing them with a wooden spoon.

4. Add the peppers, add salt and pepper, put the lid on, and cook for 20 minutes. When cooked, turn off, put the turkey and peppers on the plates, sprinkle with the cooking juices, and serve.

Turkey with Peppers (Italy)

Preparation time: 25 minutes
Cooking time: 20 minutes
Servings: 4
Calories for serving: 359

Macronutrients

- Carbs: 12 g
- Proteins: 41 g
- Fat: 9 g

Ingredients

- 28.2 oz turkey breast
- 2 yellow peppers
- 2 green peppers
- 2 carrots
- 2 stalks of celery
- 2 red onions
- Salt and pepper to taste
- Olive oil to taste

Directions

1. Wash the celery and cut it into sticks. Wash and dry the peppers and cut them into thin slices. Peel carrots and onions and cut them into slices.

2. Remove excess turkey fat and cut into cubes.

3. Heat a little oil in a pan and, when it is hot, add the vegetables and sauté for 10 minutes. After 10 minutes, add the turkey, season with salt and pepper, and cook for another 10 minutes, adding a little water if necessary.

4. When cooked, turn off and put the turkey and vegetables on the plates. Season with the cooking juices and serve.

Meat

Recipes

- Beef
- Lamb
- Pork

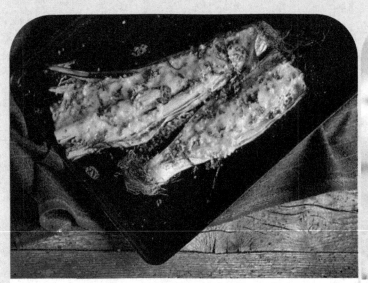

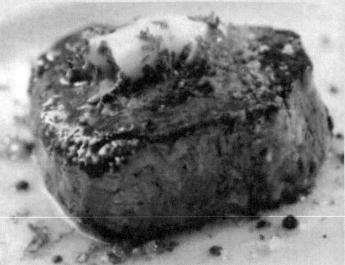

Baked Leeks and Beef (Albania)

Preparation time: 20 minutes
Cooking time: 65 minutes
Servings: 4
Calories for serving: 283

Macronutrients

- Carbs: 16 g
- Proteins: 15 g
- Fat: 8 g

Ingredients

- 35 oz leeks
- 7 oz ground beef
- ½ glass olive oil
- 1 chopped onion
- 1 tbsp ready-made tomato sauce
- Sweet red pepper to taste
- Meat broth to taste
- Salt and pepper to taste

Directions

1. Remove the green leaves of the leeks, wash them, and cut them into slices about 2.5 cm.

2. Heat some oil in a saucepan and sauté the leeks for 2 minutes. Then put the leeks in a baking pan brushed with olive oil.

3. Put the onion and the meat in the oil where you have sautéed the leeks. Add the beef broth, tomato sauce, sweet red pepper, salt, and pepper, and bring to a boil.

4. Pour the meat with all the cooking juices over the leeks and put the baking pan in the oven. Cook at 374°F for 60 minutes. Once cooked, take the baking pan out of the oven, divide the leeks into plates and serve.

Beef Fillet with Lemon (Italy)

Preparation time: 15 minutes
Cooking time: 25 minutes
Servings: 4
Calories for serving: 348

Macronutrients

- Carbs: 2 g
- Proteins: 36 g
- Fat: 9 g

Ingredients

- 21.1 oz beef tenderloin
- 1 lemon
- 1 sprig rosemary
- 1 sage leaf
- ½ glass white wine
- 1 tbsp white wine vinegar
- Salt and pepper to taste
- Olive oil to taste

Directions

1. Wash the lemon and then cut it in half. Cut one of the two halves into wedges. Wash the sage and rosemary.

2. Season the beef fillet with salt and pepper. Heat a little oil in a pan and, when it is hot, add the sage, rosemary, chopped lemon, and meat. Brown for 1 minute on each side, then add the white wine and let it evaporate.

3. Now put the lid on the pan and cook for 15 minutes, adding a little water if the bottom gets too dry. After 15 minutes, remove the aromatic herbs and lemon and blend with the vinegar and the juice of the remaining half lemon.

4. Cook for a couple of minutes, then turn off and put the meat on a cutting board. Cut the fillet into 4 smaller slices and place them on plates. Sprinkle the meat with the cooking juices and serve.

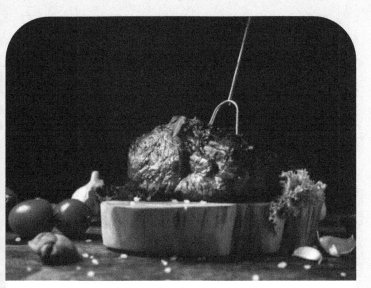

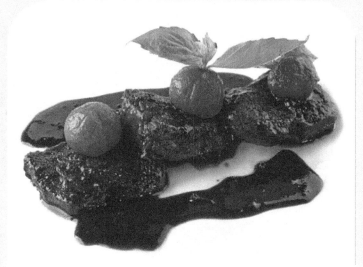

Beef Fillets with Olives (Italy)

Preparation time: 15 minutes
Cooking time: 10 minutes
Servings: 4
Calories for serving: 385

Macronutrients

- Carbs: 4 g
- Proteins: 38 g
- Fat: 10 g

Ingredients

- 4 beef fillets of 5.2 oz each
- 5.2 oz black olives
- 1 glass white wine
- Salt and pepper to taste
- Olive oil to taste

Directions

1. Remove the stone from the olives, put them in the mixer and add a drizzle of oil, salt, and pepper. Operate the mixer and blend until you get a creamy and homogeneous mixture.

2. Season the veal fillets with salt and pepper. Heat a non-stick pan and seal the fillets from all sides. Add some olive oil and cook for 2 minutes.

3. Deglaze the fillets with the white wine and let them evaporate. Remove the beef fillets from the pan and add the olives. Mix well and cook for 2 minutes.

4. Cut the fillets into thin slices and place them on plates. Sprinkle them with the olive sauce and serve.

Beef Sirloin with Balsamic Vinegar (Italy)

Preparation time: 20 minutes
Cooking time: 8 minutes
Servings: 4
Calories for serving: 332

Macronutrients

- Carbs: 2 g
- Proteins: 32 g
- Fat: 10 g

Ingredients

- 4 slices beef sirloin of 5.2 oz each
- 2 sprigs rosemary
- ½ glass balsamic vinegar
- Olive oil to taste
- Salt and pepper to taste

Directions

1. Wash the rosemary, chop it, and put it in a bowl. Add the balsamic vinegar, salt, pepper, and 4 tablespoons of olive oil. Mix well and set aside.

2. Brush the meat with olive oil and season with salt and pepper. Heat a grill and, when it is hot, put the meat to cook.

3. Cook for 4 minutes on each side, then remove the meat from the grill, put it on a chop, and cut it into slices.

4. Put the slices of meat on the plates. Sprinkle them with the balsamic vinegar sauce and serve.

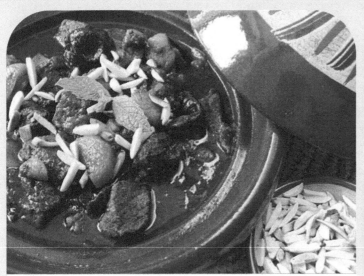

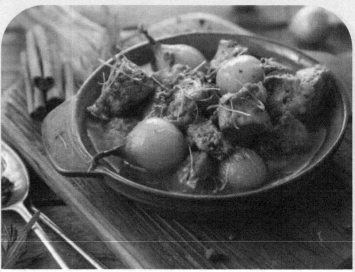

Beef with Carrots Cooked with Tajine (Morocco)

Preparation time: 20 minutes
Cooking time: 45 minutes
Servings: 4
Calories for serving: 340

Macronutrients

- Carbs: 10 g
- Proteins: 32 g
- Fat: 8 g

Ingredients

- 28.2 oz beef
- 35 oz diced carrots
- 1 clove minced garlic
- 1 tsp minced ginger
- 1 tbsp saffron
- The lemon zests
- The juice of half a lemon
- 2 tbsp green olives
- 1 tbsp chopped parsley
- Salt and pepper to taste
- Olive oil to taste

Directions

1. Cut the meat into cubes and place it in the base of the tagine with oil, garlic, ginger, saffron, and salt (you can also use a pressure cooker if you do not have the tagine). Add two glasses of water and put the lid on.

2. Cook everything for 30 minutes; then add the carrots, season with salt and pepper, sprinkle with parsley, cover, and cook for another 15–20 minutes.

3. Finally, add the zest of a lemon, the olives, and the lemon juice and reduce the sauce to an uncovered pot.

4. When the sauce has reduced, turn off, divide the meat, carrots, and olives among plates, sprinkle with the cooking juices, and serve.

Stifado (Cyprus)

Preparation time: 20 minutes
Cooking time: 35 minutes
Servings: 4
Calories for serving: 379

Macronutrients

- Carbs: 33 g
- Proteins: 34 g
- Fat: 10 g

Ingredients

- 28.2 oz beef per stew
- 28.2 oz spring onions
- 4 cloves garlic
- 5 tbsp olive oil
- 1 chopped onion
- 2 tbsp white wine vinegar
- 2 bay leaves
- 8 black peppercorns
- 1 cup tomato puree
- Salt and pepper to taste

Directions

1. Cut the meat into cubes. Heat the oil in a saucepan and fry the chopped onion. Add the meat and brown it evenly.

2. Season with salt and pepper and sprinkle with vinegar. Cover the saucepan with the lid for half a minute and then add the tomato puree, garlic, bay leaf, and black peppercorns. Then cover the meat with water and bring it to a boil.

3. Meanwhile, clean the onions, wash them under running water, and drain and salt them. Fry the onions in a pan with a drizzle of oil for a few minutes and then put them in the saucepan with the meat.

4. Cook for 15 minutes, stirring occasionally. When cooked, turn off, put the meat and onions on the plates, sprinkle with the cooking juices, and serve.

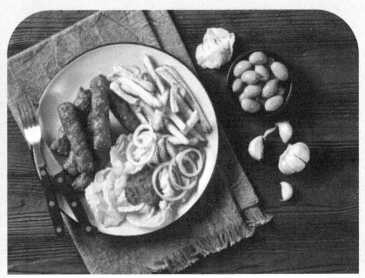

Ćevapčići (Bosnia and Herzegovina)

Preparation time: 20 minutes
Cooking time: 15 minutes
Servings: 4
Calories for serving: 296

Macronutrients

- Carbs: 2 g
- Proteins: 36 g
- Fat: 12 g

Ingredients

- 7 oz ground lamb meat
- 5.2 oz ground beef
- 5.2 oz ground pork
- 1 chopped white onion
- 1 clove minced garlic
- ½ tsp sweet paprika
- ½ tsp cumin powder
- Salt and pepper to taste
- Olive oil to taste

Directions

1. Put the 3 types of meat in a bowl and add the chopped onion and garlic. Then add the paprika, salt, pepper, and cumin and mix everything well with your hands. Cover the bowl with cling film and leave it to rest in the fridge for 2 hours.

2. After 2 hours, take the mixture from the fridge and form cylindrical meatballs about 10 cm long and 2 cm wide, working it between the palms of your hands.

3. Heat a plate and, when it is hot, put the meat to cook. Cook for 7 minutes, turning the meatballs continuously to prevent them from burning. The meatballs should be well cooked on the outside but still soft and juicy on the inside.

4. After cooking, remove the Ćevapčići from the plate, place them on plates, and serve accompanied with raw onion cut into thin slices.

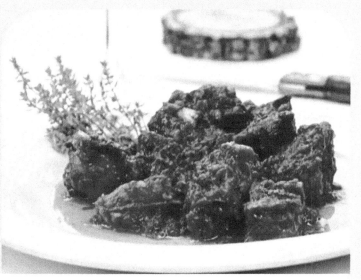

Greek-Style Lamb Stew (Greece)

Preparation time: 15 minutes + 1 hour of marinating
Cooking time: 2 hours and 10 minutes
Servings: 4
Calories for serving: 267

Macronutrients

- Carbs: 7 g
- Proteins: 33 g
- Fat: 12 g

Ingredients

- 28.2 oz lamb pulp
- 28.2 oz peeled tomato
- 1 lemon
- 1 cinnamon stick
- 1 tsp brown sugar
- Salt and pepper to taste
- Olive oil to taste

Directions

1. Cut the lamb meat into cubes and place it in a bowl. Sprinkle the meat with lemon juice and let it rest for an hour.

2. After the hour, take the meat back and put it to brown for 5 minutes in a pan with hot olive oil. After 5 minutes, add the tomato, cinnamon, and sugar.

3. Cook for 5 minutes, then season with salt and pepper, put the lid on, and continue cooking for another 2 hours.

4. After cooking, turn off and put the meat on the plates. Sprinkle it with the cooking sauce and serve.

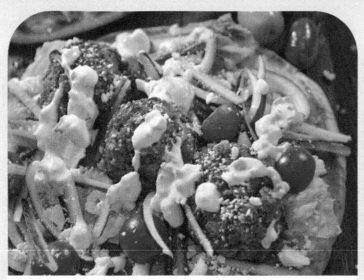

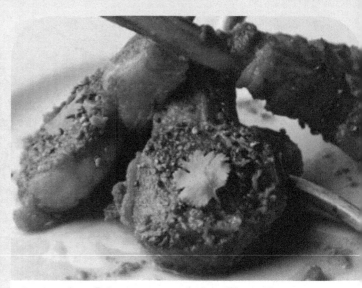

Kebab Halabi (Syria)

Preparation time: 20 minutes + 2 hours of marinating
Cooking time: 25 minutes
Servings: 4
Calories for serving: 277

Macronutrients

- Carbs: 16 g
- Proteins: 30 g
- Fat: 16 g

Ingredients

- 31.7 oz lamb pulp
- 1 white onion
- 3 tomatoes
- 4 slices Arabic bread
- 3 tsp spicy paprika
- 1 cup Greek yogurt
- 2 tbsp chopped parsley
- Salt and pepper to taste
- Olive oil to taste

Directions

1. Cut the lamb meat into cubes. Peel the onion and then chop it. Put the onion in a bowl and add the meat, paprika, salt, pepper, and 2 tablespoons of oil and leave it to marinate for at least 2 hours.

2. After 2 hours, take the meat and put it on the skewers. Heat a grill and then put the meat to cook for 15 minutes, turning it often.

3. Meanwhile, wash the tomatoes, cut them into cubes, and put them to cook in a pan with hot olive oil. Cook for 5 minutes and then add the meat marinating liquid. Cook for another 5 minutes and then turn off.

4. Heat the Arabic bread and place it on 4 plates. Pour the tomato over the slices of bread and then add the meat to the plate.

5. Mix the yogurt with oil, salt, and pepper and pour it over the meat. Sprinkle everything with the chopped parsley and serve.

Lamb Chops with Garlic (Spain)

Preparation time: 15 minutes
Cooking time: 20 minutes
Servings: 4
Calories for serving: 276

Macronutrients

- Carbs: 2 g
- Proteins: 32 g
- Fat: 14 g

Ingredients

- 28.2 oz lamb chops
- 3 cloves garlic
- 3 tbsp white wine vinegar
- ½ glass water
- ½ tsp sugar
- Salt and pepper to taste
- Olive oil to taste

Directions

1. Remove the excess fat from the chops and season with salt and pepper.

2. Heat 4 tablespoons of olive oil in a pan. When the oil is hot, add the chops and brown them for 5 minutes on each side.

3. Meanwhile, peel the garlic cloves and place them in the blender glass. Add salt, pepper, water, and vinegar and blend until you get a homogeneous mixture.

4. Pour the mixture into the pan with the meat and add the sugar. Cook for another 10 minutes, turning the meat and stirring the cooking juices from time to time.

5. Once cooked, turn off and put the chops on plates. Season the meat with the cooking juices and serve.

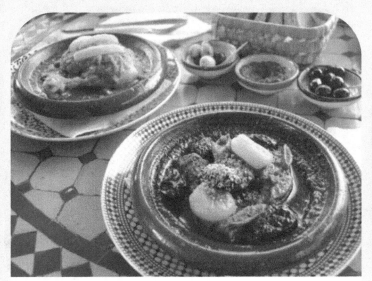

Lamb Tajine with Plums (Morocco)

Preparation time: 20 minutes
Cooking time: 1 hour and 50 minutes
Servings: 4
Calories for serving: 429

Macronutrients

- Carbs: 18 g
- Proteins: 37 g
- Fat: 15 g

Ingredients

- 24.9 oz lamb shoulder
- 7 oz prunes
- 1 tsp ginger
- 2 clove garlic, minced
- 1 tbsp sugar
- 1 onion
- 1 piece cinnamon stick
- 1 tsp saffron
- 1 tbsp sesame
- 1.7 oz peeled almonds
- Salt and pepper to taste
- Olive oil to taste

Directions

1. Put the prunes in a saucepan with warm water and let them soften for 30 minutes.

2. After 30 minutes, add the cinnamon and sugar and simmer for 10 minutes.

3. Peel the garlic and onion, chop them, and fry them in a saucepan that can also go in the oven with 5 tablespoons of oil, ginger, and saffron, or, if you have it, you can use the tajine.

4. Cut the lamb into cubes and place it in the saucepan. Brown it for 10 minutes, stirring constantly. Now add the plums with the cooking liquid, season with salt and pepper, and place the covered saucepan, with a lid or with aluminum foil, in the oven to cook for 1 hour and 30 minutes at 356°F.

5. Meanwhile, toast the sesame seeds and almonds in a non-stick pan.

6. After cooking, remove the saucepan from the oven. Put the meat, plums, and cooking juices on the plates. Sprinkle with almonds and sesame seeds and serve.

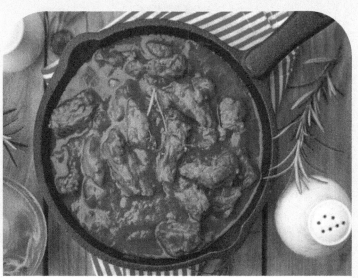

Tas Kempap, Lamb Chops with Tomato Sauce (Greece)

Preparation time: 20 minutes
Cooking time: 75 minutes
Servings: 4
Calories for serving: 422

Macronutrients

- Carbs: 5 g
- Proteins: 46 g
- Fat: 18 g

Ingredients

- 28.2 oz lamb meat
- 17.6 oz onions
- 1 cup peeled tomatoes
- ½ glass white wine
- Chopped parsley to taste
- Salt and pepper to taste
- Olive oil to taste

Directions

1. Cut the meat into medium-sized cubes. Peel the onions and cut them into slices.

2. Put some oil in a pan and let it heat up. When it is hot, add the meat and brown it for 5 minutes, turning it often. After 5 minutes, add the onions.

3. Sauté for a couple of minutes, then add the white wine and let it evaporate. Add the peeled tomatoes and season with salt and pepper and add the parsley. Mix well and cook for 60 minutes, stirring occasionally and adding water if the cooking juices dry out too much.

4. After cooking, turn off, put the meat and the cooking juices on the plates, and serve.

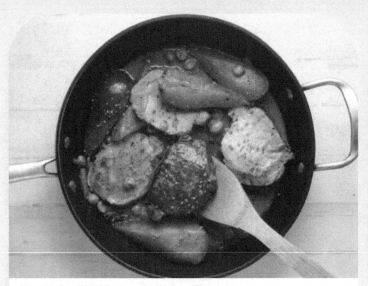

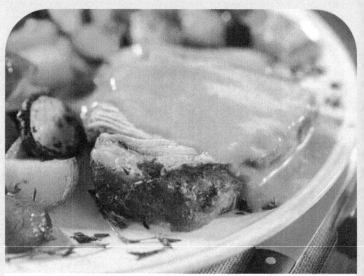

Pork Fillet with Pears

Preparation time: 20 minutes
Cooking time: 35 minutes
Servings: 4
Calories for serving: 420

Macronutrients

- Carbs: 16 g
- Proteins: 44 g
- Fat: 18 g

Ingredients

- 28.2 oz pork tenderloin
- 14 oz pears
- 1 glass apple cider vinegar
- 1 onion
- 1 sprig rosemary
- Olive oil to taste
- Salt and pepper to taste

Directions

1. Wash the rosemary. Remove the excess fat from the meat and then tie it with kitchen twine. Put the rosemary between the string and the meat.

2. Peel the onion and cut it into thin slices. Peel the pears, remove the seeds, and then cut them into cubes.

3. Heat some oil in a pan and add the onion and pears. Mix well and cook for 2 minutes, then add the meat. Brown the meat on all sides, then add the apple cider vinegar.

4. Lower the heat, season with salt and pepper, and cook for 25 minutes. After 25 minutes, remove the meat from the pan and cut it into slices. Take an immersion blender and blend the pears and the cooking juices, until you get a smooth and homogeneous sauce.

5. Put the pork slices on plates, sprinkle with the pear sauce and serve.

Pork Fillet with Walnuts (Italy)

Preparation time: 15 minutes
Cooking time: 30 minutes
Servings: 4
Calories for serving: 406

Macronutrients

- Carbs: 12 g
- Proteins: 33 g
- Fat: 16 g

Ingredients

- 17.6 oz pork tenderloin
- 2.4 oz chopped walnuts
- 1 and a half cup milk
- 1 tsp corn starch
- Salt and pepper to taste
- Olive oil to taste

Directions

1. Put 4 tablespoons of olive oil in a pan and let it heat up. Put the fillet in the pan and brown it on all sides.

2. Meanwhile, put the walnuts and milk in a saucepan and heat up. When the milk is hot, pour it into the pan with the pork. Season with salt and pepper and cook for 15 minutes.

3. After 15 minutes, take the meat, put it wrapped in a sheet of aluminum foil, and temporarily set it aside.

4. Meanwhile, take an immersion blender, blend the cooking juices, and let it thicken for a few minutes.

5. Now put the meat on a cutting board and cut it into slices. Put the pork slices on a plate, sprinkle with the walnut sauce and serve.

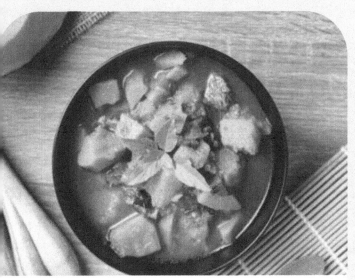

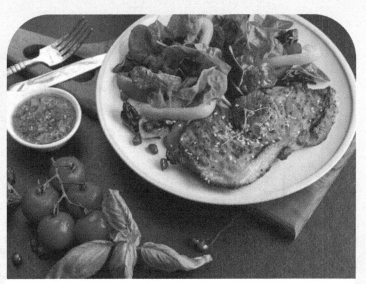

Pork Stew with Pumpkin (Italy)

Preparation time: 20 minutes
Cooking time: 60 minutes
Servings: 4
Calories for serving: 416

Macronutrients

- Carbs: 11 g
- Proteins: 36 g
- Fat: 15 g

Ingredients

- 21 oz pork shoulder
- 14 oz pumpkin pulp
- 1 and a half cup meat broth
- 1 glass red wine
- 1 minced clove garlic
- 2 sage leaves
- 1 sprig rosemary
- Flour to taste
- Salt and pepper to taste
- Olive oil to taste

Directions

1. Cut the pork into cubes. Put the flour on a plate, add salt and pepper, and mix. Dip the pork cubes in flour and flour them well on all sides.

2. Put the meat in a pan with hot olive oil and brown it well. Add the wine and let it evaporate.

3. Now add the sage and rosemary, and a cup of broth, put the lid on and cook for 30 minutes.

4. Meanwhile, wash the pumpkin pulp and cut it into cubes. After 30 minutes, add the pumpkin, season with salt and pepper, and add the remaining broth.

5. After cooking, turn off and put the meat and pumpkin on the plates. Sprinkle with the cooking juices and serve.

Pork with Peppers (Italy)

Preparation time: 20 minutes
Cooking time: 55 minutes
Servings: 4
Calories for serving: 384

Macronutrients

- Carbs: 10 g
- Proteins: 39 g
- Fat: 15 g

Ingredients

- 24.6 oz pork loin
- 3.5 oz yellow peppers
- 3.5 oz red peppers
- 5.2 oz tomatoes
- ½ glass white wine
- ½ glass water
- 1 clove minced garlic
- Salt and pepper to taste
- Olive oil to taste

Directions

1. Wash the peppers, remove the seeds, and cut them into strips. Wash the tomatoes and then cut them into cubes.

2. Meanwhile, put some oil to heat in a pan and, when it is hot, add the garlic and brown it. Now add the meat and brown it for 5 minutes.

3. After 5 minutes, blend with the wine and let it evaporate. Now add the peppers, tomatoes, salt, and pepper and mix well. Add the water, put the lid on, and cook for 40 minutes.

4. Once cooked, remove the meat, and place it on a cutting board. Blend the cooking juices with an immersion blender. Cut the meat into slices and place it on plates. Sprinkle with the blended cooking juices and serve.

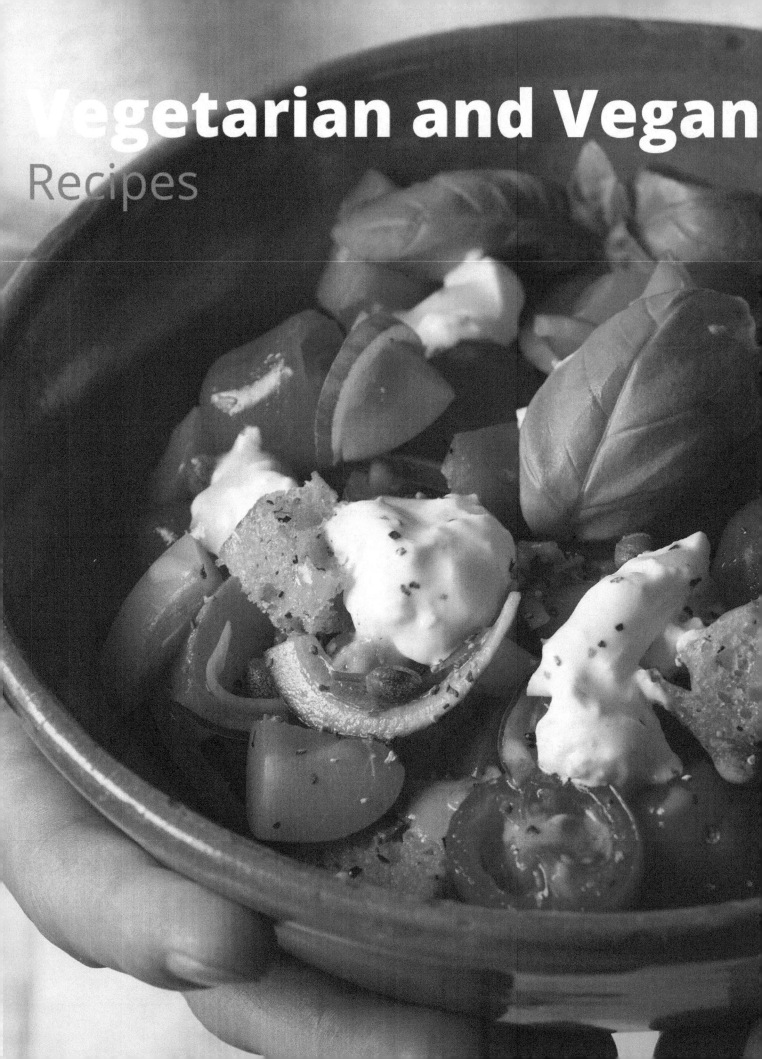

Vegetarian and Vegan

Recipes

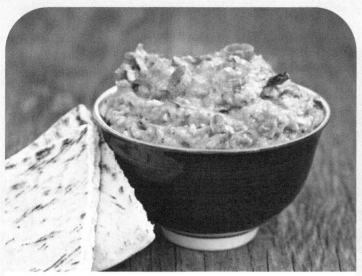

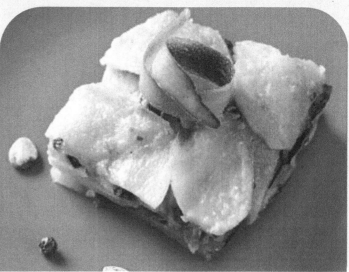

Babaganoush (Lebanon)

Preparation time: 25 minutes
Cooking time: 30 minutes
Servings: 4
Calories for serving: 107

Macronutrients

- Carbs: 14 g
- Proteins: 4 g
- Fat: 7 g

Ingredients

- 4 eggplants
- 3 tbsp Tahini
- 2 tbsp lemon juice
- 1 clove minced garlic
- 4 tbsp Greek yogurt
- Salt and pepper to taste
- Olive oil to taste

Directions

1. Wash the eggplants and cut them in half. With a knife make incisions along the part of the pulp. Season with oil, salt, and pepper and fold the two halves on themselves and wrap them in aluminum foil.

2. Bake the eggplants in the oven at 392°F for 15 minutes. After 15 minutes, open the aluminum paper and cook the eggplants until the peel is almost black.

3. Once cooked, remove the eggplants from the oven, place them on a cutting board and let them cool.

4. Meanwhile, in a bowl, mix the garlic, lemon juice, yogurt, salt, and pepper. Remove the pulp from the eggplants with a spoon and pour it into the bowl with the sauce, mashing everything well with a fork. Stir until you get a homogeneous and creamy mixture.

5. When the mixture is ready, add the Tahini and mix again. Serve in a bowl accompanied with Arabic bread.

Briam with Potatoes and Zucchinis (Greece)

Preparation time: 25 minutes
Cooking time: 1 hour
Servings: 4
Calories for serving: 268

Macronutrients

- Carbs: 36 g
- Proteins: 10 g
- Fat: 9 g

Ingredients

- 28.2 oz potatoes
- 28.2 oz zucchinis
- 17.6 oz tomatoes
- 3 minced garlic cloves
- Chopped parsley to taste
- Salt and pepper to taste
- Olive oil to taste

Directions

1. Peel the potatoes, wash them, and then cut them into slices. Peel the zucchinis, wash them, and then cut them into thin slices lengthwise. Wash the tomatoes, peel them, and then cut them into cubes.

2. Brush a baking pan with olive oil and put a layer of zucchinis on the bottom. Season with oil, salt, and pepper, and sprinkle with a little parsley and minced garlic.

3. Pour over half of the tomatoes, and then put the potatoes. Season with salt and pepper and repeat the same operation until the end of the ingredients.

4. Now pour over ½ glass of oil and 3 cups of water and put the baking pan in the oven. Cook at 356°F for 1 hour. After cooking, remove the baking pan from the oven. Divide the briam into 4 parts, put it on serving plates and serve.

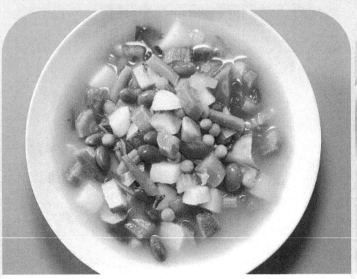 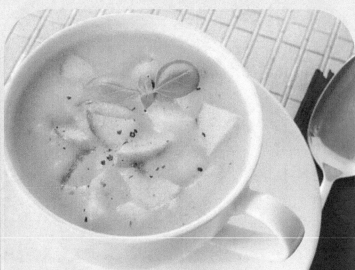

Chortosoupa - Vegetable Soup (Greece)

Preparation time: 25 minutes
Cooking time: 35 minutes
Servings: 4
Calories for serving: 102

Macronutrients

- Carbs: 35 g
- Proteins: 2 g
- Fat: 6 g

Ingredients

- 3 potatoes
- 3 carrots
- 1 white onion
- 2 stalks of celery
- 2 zucchinis
- 2 ripe red tomatoes
- Grated lemon zest to taste
- Olive oil to taste
- Salt and pepper to taste

Directions

1. Peel the potatoes, zucchinis, and carrots, wash them, and then cut them into cubes. Peel the onion and then cut it into slices. Wash the tomatoes and then cut them into cubes. Peel the celery and then chop it.

2. Heat a little oil in a saucepan and, when it is hot, put all the vegetables inside. Season with salt and pepper, stir and cook for 2 minutes.

3. Now cover the vegetables with water and cook for 25 minutes.

4. After cooking, put the soup on plates, season with a little oil, sprinkle with lemon zest, and serve.

Croatian Apple Soup (Croatia)

Preparation time: 20 minutes
Cooking time: 20 minutes
Servings: 4
Calories for serving: 270

Macronutrients

- Carbs: 20 g
- Proteins: 5 g
- Fat: 10 g

Ingredients

- 6 yellow apples
- 1 tsp cinnamon powder
- ½ lemon
- 2 cups water
- 1 tbsp flour
- ½ glass white wine
- 1 tbsp sugar
- ½ cup toasted croutons
- Salt and pepper to taste
- Olive oil to taste

Directions

1. Peel the apples and quarter them, removing the cores, then cut the pulp into cubes.

2. Put the apples in a saucepan, add the cinnamon, and lemon juice, cover them with water and let everything cook until the apples are almost pulped.

3. Once cooked, pass the apples through a sieve, and collect the pulp in a bowl.

4. Meanwhile, heat two tablespoons of oil in a saucepan, add the flour and let it toast for a few seconds, stirring constantly. Then blend with the wine and continue mixing. Add the sugar, and apple purée and let it boil for a minute.

5. Turn off and put the soup on the plates. Add the croutons and serve.

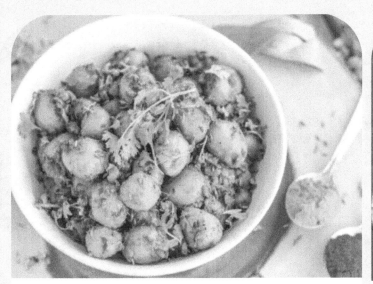

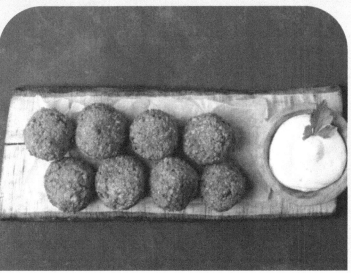

Cumin Potatoes (Tunisia)

Preparation time: 20 minutes
Cooking time: 15 minutes
Servings: 4
Calories for serving: 375

Macronutrients

- Carbs: 40 g
- Proteins: 10 g
- Fat: 10 g

Ingredients

- 28.2 oz potatoes
- 2 tbsp cumin
- 4 tbsp harissa sauce
- 1 lemon juice
- 1 tbsp chopped parsley
- Salt and pepper to taste
- Olive oil to taste

Directions

1. Peel the potatoes, wash them, and cut them into pieces of about 2.5 cm. Put them in a pot with water and salt and let them boil for 15 minutes. Once cooked, drain, and let them cool in a bowl.

2. In a small bowl, mix the cumin, Harissa sauce, lemon juice, and 3 tablespoons of oil.

3. Season the cold potatoes with the cumin mixture, season with salt and pepper, and mix everything well.

4. Sprinkle with chopped parsley, put the potatoes on plates and serve.

Falafel (Palestine)

Preparation time: 20 minutes + 1 hour of rest
Cooking time: 10 minutes
Servings: 4
Calories for serving: 595

Macronutrients

- Carbs: 69 g
- Proteins: 27 g
- Fat: 15 g

Ingredients

- 17.6 oz cooked chickpeas
- 1 onion
- 1 clove garlic
- 2 tbsp chopped parsley
- Cumin powder to taste
- Salt and pepper to taste
- Olive oil to taste

Directions

1. Peel the onion and then cut it into pieces. Peel the garlic and put it in the mixer together with the onion. Then add the chickpeas, salt, pepper, and cumin.

2. Operate the mixer and chop until you get a homogeneous and thick mixture. Put the mixture in a bowl, add the parsley and mix well.

3. Cover the bowl with cling film and leave it to rest in the fridge for 1 hour. After the hour, resume the mixture and form round meatballs which you will then crush with your hands.

4. Put the falafel in a baking pan brushed with olive oil and sprinkle a little oil on the surface. Place the baking pan in the oven and cook for 10 minutes at 392°F.

5. Once cooked, place the still hot falafel on serving plates and serve.

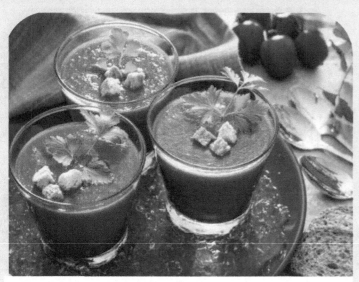

Gazpacho (Spain)

Preparation time: 40 minutes
Servings: 4
Calories for serving: 102

Macronutrients

- Carbs: 16 g
- Proteins: 2 g
- Fat: 5 g

Ingredients

- 35 oz ripe tomatoes
- 2.8 oz green peppers
- 8.8 oz cucumbers
- 3.5 oz onions
- 1 clove
- ½ glass vinegar
- 2.1 oz stale bread
- Salt and pepper to taste
- Olive oil to taste

Directions

1. Break up the bread and put it to soak in cold water. Wash the tomatoes, cut them in half, and remove the pulp and seeds. Put the pulp and seeds of the tomatoes in a bowl. Peel the onion and then cut it into slices. Wash the cucumber and cut it into cubes.

2. Cut the garlic into two parts and remove the internal germ. Put the vegetables and garlic in a bowl, add the squeezed bread, add salt, and pepper and mix well. Set aside and marinate for 10 minutes.

3. After 10 minutes, add the vinegar to the vegetables and blend everything with an immersion blender. Blend until you get a creamy and homogeneous mixture.

4. Now pour the gazpacho into 4 soup plates, season with a little oil and pepper, and serve.

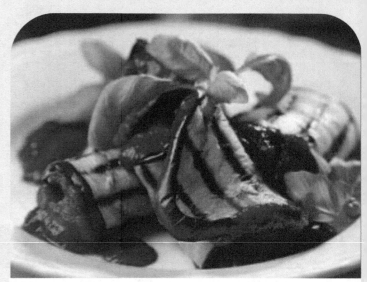

Mediterranean-Style Eggplant Rolls (Italy)

Preparation time: 20 minutes
Cooking time: 35 minutes
Servings: 4
Calories for serving: 226

Macronutrients

- Carbs: 9 g
- Proteins: 7 g
- Fat: 10 g

Ingredients

- 4.2 oz eggplant
- 3.5 oz mozzarella
- 7 oz tomato puree
- 1 tbsp black olives
- 4 basil leaves
- 1 minced clove
- Salt and pepper to taste
- Olive oil to taste

Directions

1. Heat a little oil in a saucepan, add the garlic and brown it. Add the tomato puree, season with salt and pepper, and cook for 15 minutes.

2. Meanwhile, wash the eggplant and cut it into slices about 1 cm thick. Heat a grill and, as soon as it is hot, put the eggplants on the grill. Once cooked, put the eggplants on a cutting board and season with oil, salt, and pepper.

3. When the sauce is ready, turn it off and brush the eggplants with the sauce. Cut the olives into pieces and the mozzarella into thin slices. Put the mozzarella on top of the sauce, then some olives, and finally the basil.

4. Roll the eggplants on themselves and place them in a small baking dish with the closure facing down. Finally, cover the rolls with a little tomato sauce and put the baking dish in the oven. Cook at 356°F for 10 minutes.

5. Once cooked, remove the baking dish from the oven, place the eggplant rolls on the plates and serve.

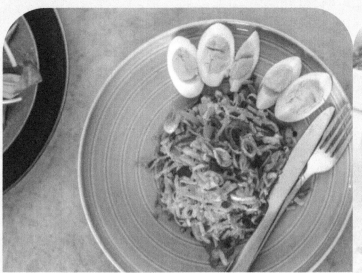

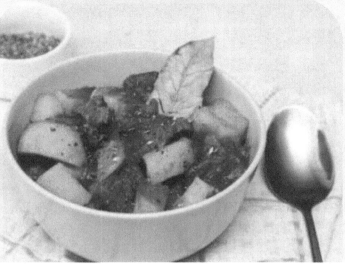

Omek Houria (Tunisia)

Preparation time: 20 minutes+ 1 hour of rest
Cooking time: 30 minutes
Servings: 4
Calories for serving: 150

Macronutrients

- Carbs: 25 g
- Proteins: 10 g
- Fat: 10 g

Ingredients

- 2 carrots
- 1 hard-boiled egg
- 2 potatoes
- 1 tsp harissa sauce
- 6 black olives
- 6 green olives
- 1 tbsp chopped parsley
- Salt and pepper to taste
- Olive oil to taste

Directions

1. Peel the potatoes and carrots, wash them, cut them into cubes, and then boil them in plenty of salted water. Cook for 30 minutes, then drain and let them cool.

2. Shell the hard-boiled egg, cut it into small pieces and put it in a bowl. Add the carrots and potatoes and mix.

3. Dilute the harissa sauce with a tablespoon of oil and a drop of water and then put it in the bowl with the vegetables.

4. Season with a little more oil, salt, and pepper and put in the fridge to rest for 1 hour.

5. After the hour, take the vegetables from the fridge, add the olives and parsley, mix, then divide into plates and serve.

Potatoes with Tomato Sauce (Greece)

Preparation time: 20 minutes
Cooking time: 30 minutes
Servings: 4
Calories for serving: 234

Macronutrients

- Carbs: 30 g
- Proteins: 4 g
- Fat: 6 g

Ingredients

- 28.2 oz potatoes
- ½ onion
- 21.1 oz tomato puree
- 1 tbsp chopped parsley
- Dried oregano to taste
- Salt and pepper to taste
- Olive oil to taste

Directions

1. Peel and wash the potatoes. Then cut them into pieces that are not too small.

2. Peel the onion and then chop it. Heat some oil in a saucepan and then put the onion to sauté for 3 minutes. Then add the tomato puree and season with salt and pepper. Boil and then add the potatoes and sprinkle with oregano.

3. Cook for a couple of minutes and then add 3 cups of water. Cook for another 25 minutes or until the potatoes are soft.

4. Once cooked, put the potatoes and the sauce on the plates, sprinkle with the chopped parsley, and serve.

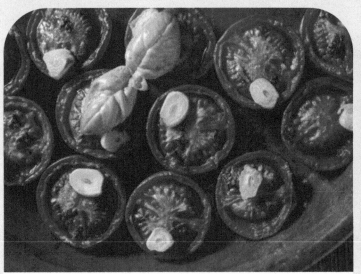

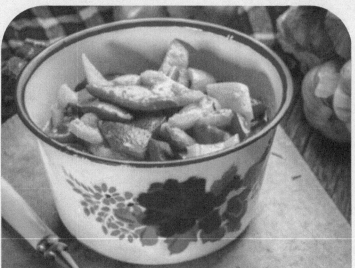

Roasted Tomatoes (Italy)

Preparation time: 20 minutes
Cooking time: 10 minutes
Servings: 4
Calories for serving: 114

Macronutrients

- Carbs: 14 g
- Proteins: 4 g
- Fat: 4 g

Ingredients

- 35 oz ripe red tomatoes
- 3 minced garlic cloves
- Chopped parsley to taste
- Salt and pepper to taste
- Olive oil to taste

Directions

1. Wash and dry the tomatoes and remove the cap.

2. Brush a baking pan with olive oil and place the tomatoes inside with the cap side facing up.

3. Put the garlic cloves, and parsley in a bowl and add salt, pepper, and olive oil. Mix well and then pour the mixture over the tomatoes.

4. Place the baking pan in the oven and bake at 356°F for 10 minutes. Once cooked, take the baking pan out of the oven, put the tomatoes on serving plates, and serve.

Stewed Peppers (Italy)

Preparation time: 20 minutes
Cooking time: 45 minutes
Servings: 4
Calories for serving: 120

Macronutrients

- Carbs: 21 g
- Proteins: 5 g
- Fat: 13 g

Ingredients

- 2 red peppers
- 1 yellow pepper
- 3 tomatoes
- 1 red onion
- 1 clove garlic, minced
- Salt and pepper to taste
- Olive oil to taste

Directions

1. Wash and dry the peppers, remove the cap and seeds, and then cut them into slices that are not too thin.

2. Boil some water with salt and then pour it into a bowl. Add the tomatoes, keep them immersed for 30 seconds, then peel them and cut them into cubes. Peel the onion and then cut it into slices.

3. Heat a little oil in a pan and then add the onion and garlic and sauté for 3 minutes. After 3 minutes, add the tomatoes and peppers, season with salt and pepper, and mix well.

4. Cook for 20 minutes, with the lid on, and stirring occasionally. After 20 minutes, remove the lid and cook for another 20 minutes, adding a little water if the bottom dries too much.

5. After cooking, turn off, put the peppers and the cooking juices on the plates, and serve.

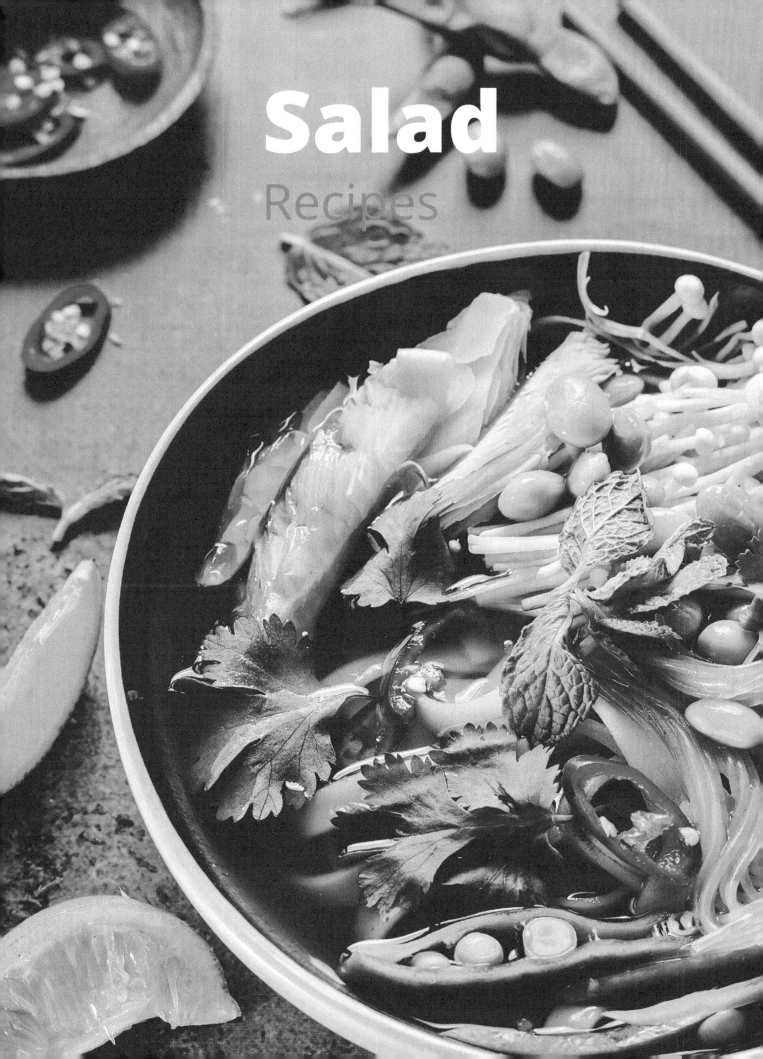

Salad

Recipes

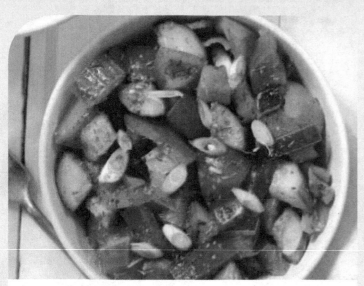

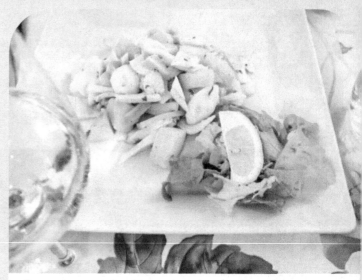

Baladi (Egypt)

Preparation time: 15 minutes
Servings: 4
Calories for serving: 210

Macronutrients

- Carbs: 21 g
- Proteins: 3 g
- Fat: 3 g

Ingredients

- 4 ripe red tomatoes
- 2 red onions
- 2 cucumbers
- 1 red pepper
- 1 tbsp chopped parsley
- 2 tbsp vinegar
- 1 lemon
- Olive oil to taste
- Salt and pepper to taste

Directions

1. Wash and dry the tomatoes and then cut them into cubes. Peel the cucumbers and cut them into cubes. Peel the onions and cut them into slices. Wash the pepper and cut it into cubes.

2. Put the vegetables in a bowl and add the parsley. Season with oil, salt, pepper, vinegar, and lemon juice.

3. Mix well and serve.

Calamari, Potato, and Celery Salad (Italy)

Preparation time: 25 minutes
Cooking time: 45 minutes
Servings: 4
Calories for serving: 250

Macronutrients

- Carbs: 21 g
- Proteins: 30 g
- Fat: 8 g

Ingredients

- 24.6 oz pre-cleaned squid
- 17.6 oz potatoes
- 2 stalks of celery
- 1 lime
- Chopped parsley to taste
- Salt and pepper to taste
- Olive oil to taste

Directions

1. Wash the potatoes with all the peel, put them in a pot full of water and salt, and cook for 40 minutes. Once cooked, drain the potatoes, pass them under cold water, then peel them and cut them into cubes.

2. Wash the squid, then put them in a pot with boiling water and salt and cook for 10 minutes. After cooking, drain the squid, let them cool, and then cut them into rings.

3. Wash and cut the celery stalks into small pieces and put them in a bowl. Add the squid and potatoes.

4. Put the lime juice, salt, pepper, and oil in a bowl and mix well. Pour the emulsion into the bowl with the squid. Stir, then put the bowl on the table and serve.

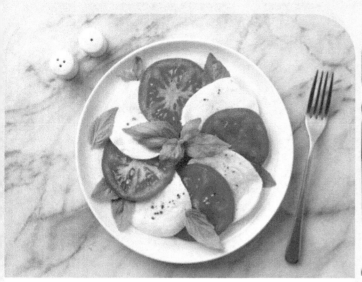 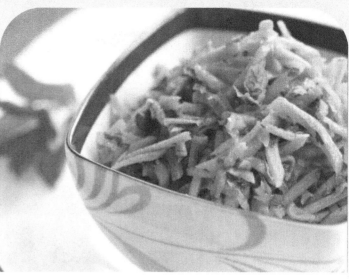

Caprese Salad (Italy)

Preparation time: 15 minutes
Servings: 4
Calories for serving: 369

Macronutrients

- Carbs: 10 g
- Proteins: 32 g
- Fat: 23 g

Ingredients

- 17.6 oz mozzarella
- 14 of tomatoes
- 8 basil leaves
- Salt and pepper to taste
- Olive oil to taste

Directions

1. Wash and dry the tomatoes. Cut the tomatoes into thin slices.

2. Cut the mozzarella into slices.

3. Arrange the slices of mozzarella and tomato on a plate. Arrange them in the shape of a circle, alternating the tomato with the mozzarella.

4. Season with oil, salt, and pepper. Add the chopped basil leaves, put the dish on the table and serve.

Carrot, Onion, and Lemon Salad (Italy)

Preparation time: 20 minutes+ 15 minutes to rest
Servings: 4
Calories for serving: 94

Macronutrients

- Carbs: 16 g
- Proteins: 2 g
- Fat: 4 g

Ingredients

- 4 carrots
- 1 lemon
- 1 red onion
- Chopped dill to taste
- Salt and pepper to taste
- Olive oil to taste

Directions

1. Wash and scrub the carrots well to remove all earthy residues. Cut the carrots into thin slices lengthwise and place them in a bowl.

2. Peel the onion, chop it and pour it into the bowl with the carrots.

3. Put the lemon juice, salt, pepper, and oil in a bowl and sprinkle the carrots and onion on top.

4. Add the dill and mix well. Cook for 15 minutes, then put the salad on the table and serve.

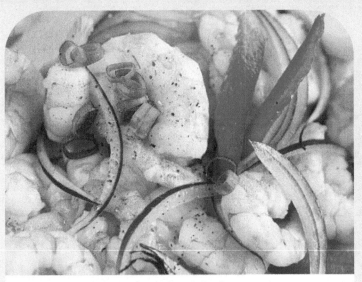

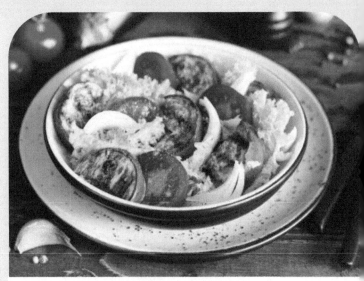

Catalan Salad (Spain)

Preparation time: 20 minutes
Cooking time: 42 minutes
Servings: 4
Calories for serving: 217

Macronutrients

- Carbs: 22 g
- Proteins: 18 g
- Fat: 7 g

Ingredients

- 12.3 oz potatoes
- 7 oz cherry tomatoes
- 12 shrimps
- 1 red onion
- 1 tbsp grain mustard
- 1 tbsp vinegar
- Chopped parsley to taste
- Salt and pepper to taste

Directions

1. Wash the potatoes thoroughly under running water, then put them in a saucepan, add a tablespoon of salt and cover with cold water. Cook for about 40 minutes. After 40 minutes, drain the potatoes, pass them under cold water, peel them, and then cut them into slices.

2. Wash the cherry tomatoes and cut them into 4 wedges. Peel the onion and cut it into slices.

3. Shell the shrimps, remove the intestinal filament, wash them, and pat them with a paper towel. Put a pot of water and salt on the heat and, as soon as it starts to boil, put the shrimps, and cook for 2 minutes. Once cooked, drain the shrimp, and let them cool.

4. Meanwhile, put the mustard, vinegar, salt, pepper, and olive oil in a bowl and mix until a smooth sauce is obtained.

5. Now put the shrimp, potatoes, onion, and cherry tomatoes in a bowl, toss with the mustard sauce and mix well. Sprinkle with chopped parsley and serve.

Eggplant Salad (Greece)

Preparation time: 20 minutes
Cooking time: 60 minutes
Servings: 4
Calories for serving: 221

Macronutrients

- Carbs: 19 g
- Proteins: 7 g
- Fat: 9 g

Ingredients

- 4 eggplants
- 2 tomatoes
- 1 onion
- 1 lemon
- 1 tbsp chopped parsley
- Salt and pepper to taste
- Olive oil to taste

Directions

1. Remove the cap from the eggplants. Wash them, prick them with the tines of a fork, and put them in the oven. Cook at 356°F for 1 hour.

2. Once cooked, take the eggplants out of the oven, cut them in half, and remove the pulp by digging them out with a spoon. Squeeze the pulp of the eggplant well to remove as much liquid as possible, then chop the pulp coarsely and put it in a bowl.

3. Peel the onion, cut it into slices, and put it in the bowl with the pulp of the eggplant. Wash the tomatoes, cut them into cubes, and put them in the bowl with the rest of the ingredients.

4. Season everything with oil, salt, pepper, and lemon juice, and sprinkle with chopped parsley. Mix well and then serve.

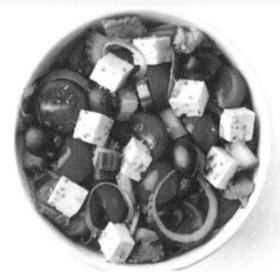

Onion and Feta Salad (Greece)

Preparation time: 20 minutes
Servings: 4
Calories for serving: 194

Macronutrients

- Carbs: 8 g
- Proteins: 9 g
- Fat: 14 g

Ingredients

- 10.5 oz tomatoes
- 1 large onion
- 1 cucumber
- 5.2 oz feta
- 12 black olives
- Dried oregano to taste
- 1 tbsp white wine vinegar
- Salt and pepper to taste
- Olive oil to taste

Directions

1. Wash the tomatoes and cut them into cubes. Peel the cucumber, wash it and cut it into cubes. Peel the onion and then cut it into slices. Cut the feta into cubes.

2. Put all the ingredients in a bowl.

3. Put the oil, vinegar, oregano, salt, and pepper in another bowl and mix well.

4. Add the olives to the bowl dressed with the vinaigrette, mix well and then serve.

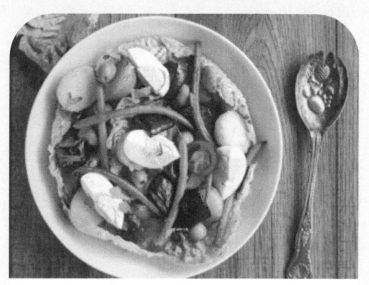

Potato, Green Beans, and Egg Salad (Italy)

Preparation time: 20 minutes
Cooking time: 15 minutes
Servings: 4
Calories for serving: 226

Macronutrients

- Carbs: 19 g
- Proteins: 8 g
- Fat: 9 g

Ingredients

- 17.6 oz potatoes
- 10.5 oz green beans
- 2 hard-boiled eggs
- 1 clove minced garlic
- 1 lemon
- Chopped parsley to taste
- Salt and pepper to taste
- Olive oil to taste

Directions

1. Peel the potatoes, wash them, and then cut them into cubes. Put them in a pot with salted boiling water and cook for 15 minutes.

2. Check the green beans, wash them, and then put them to cook in a pot with boiling salted water for 15 minutes. After cooking, turn off, drain the potatoes, and green beans and let them cool.

3. Meanwhile, put the oil, salt, pepper, garlic, lemon juice, and parsley in a bowl and mix well.

4. Peel the eggs, cut them into wedges, and put them in a salad bowl. Add the potatoes and green beans.

5. Sprinkle with the lemon and parsley emulsion and mix well. Put the salad bowl on the table and serve.

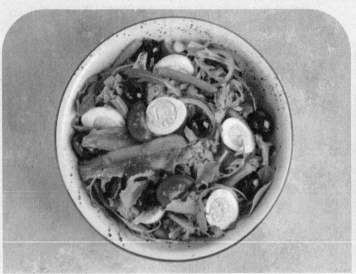

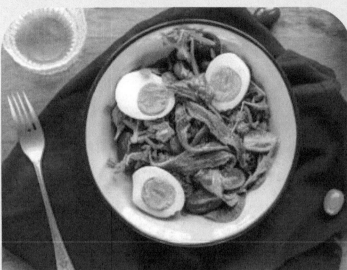

Salade Nicoise (French Riviera, France)

Preparation time: 20 minutes
Cooking time: 15 minutes
Servings: 4
Calories for serving: 405

Macronutrients

- Carbs: 12 g
- Proteins: 32 g
- Fat: 12 g

Ingredients

- 2 potatoes
- 7 oz green beans
- 3 tomatoes
- 6 anchovies in oil
- 3.5 oz black olives
- 3.5 oz tuna in oil
- ½ red onion
- 2 hard-boiled eggs
- ½ red pepper
- 6 lettuce leaves
- Vinegar to taste
- Salt and pepper to taste
- Olive oil to taste

Directions

1. Check the green beans and put them to boil in salted boiling water for 15 minutes. Peel the potatoes, cut them into cubes and boil them in boiling salted water for 15 minutes. When the potatoes and green beans are cooked, drain and let them cool.

2. Wash and dry the lettuce leaves and then cut them into small pieces. Wash the tomatoes and then cut them into slices. Peel the onion and cut it into thin slices. Wash the pepper and then cut it into slices.

3. Put the potatoes, green beans cut in half, lettuce, onion, and tomatoes in a bowl.

4. Peel the eggs and then cut them into 4 wedges. Put the eggs in the bowl with the vegetables along with the tuna and drained anchovies.

5. Finally, add the black olives, season with salt, pepper, oil, and vinegar, mix well and then serve.

Salad with Eggs and Anchovies (Algeria)

Preparation time: 20 minutes
Servings: 4
Calories for serving: 210

Macronutrients

- Carbs: 20 g
- Proteins: 8 g
- Fat: 12 g

Ingredients

- 2 red peppers
- 4 medium ripe tomatoes
- 1.7 oz cucumber
- 2 onions
- 4.2 oz black olives
- 6 chopped anchovy fillets
- 2 hard-boiled eggs
- 1 tsp chopped fresh basil
- 1 tbsp vinegar
- Salt and pepper to taste
- Olive oil to taste

Directions

1. Wash the peppers, tomatoes, and cucumber, and then cut them into cubes. Peel the onions and then cut them into slices.

2. Cut the hard-boiled eggs into 8 wedges.

3. Now put all the ingredients in a bowl.

4. Season with oil, salt, pepper and vinegar, mix well and serve.

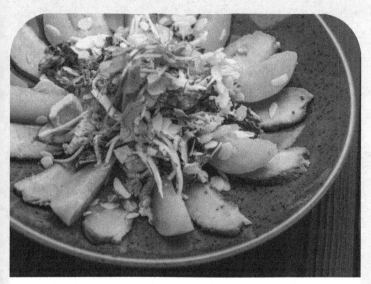
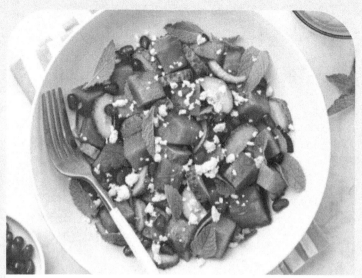

Tuna and Citrus Salad (Italy)

Preparation time: 20 minutes
Cooking time: 8 minutes
Servings: 4
Calories for serving: 238

Macronutrients

- Carbs: 10 g
- Proteins: 20 g
- Fat: 6 g

Ingredients

- 14 oz tuna fillet
- 2 oranges
- 1 lemon
- ½ fennel
- Olive oil to taste
- Salt and pepper to taste

Directions

1. Brush the tuna with olive oil and season with salt and pepper. Heat a grill and cook for 2 minutes on each side. Once cooked, put the tuna on a cutting board and cut it into slices.

2. Peel the oranges and lemon taking care to remove all the white part that covers the pulp with a knife and then cut them into cubes.

3. Wash the fennel, remove the hardest leaves, and then cut it into slices.

4. Put the citrus pulp, fennel, and finally the slices of tuna in a serving dish. Season with oil, salt, and pepper, cook for 5 minutes, then put on the table and serve.

Watermelon and Cucumber Salad (Greece)

Preparation time: 15 minutes
Servings: 4
Calories for serving: 190

Macronutrients

- Carbs: 14 g
- Proteins: 6 g
- Fat: 13 g

Ingredients

- 17.6 oz watermelon
- 2 cucumbers
- ½ onions
- 8.8 oz feta
- Mint to taste
- Salt and pepper to taste
- Olive oil to taste

Directions

1. Remove the ends from the cucumbers, wash them, and then cut them into slices. Remove the skin and seeds from the watermelon and then cut them into cubes. Peel the onion and then cut it into thin slices.

2. Put all the ingredients in a bowl and add the crumbled feta and chopped mint leaves.

3. Season with oil, salt, and pepper. Mix well and serve.

Dessert

Recipes

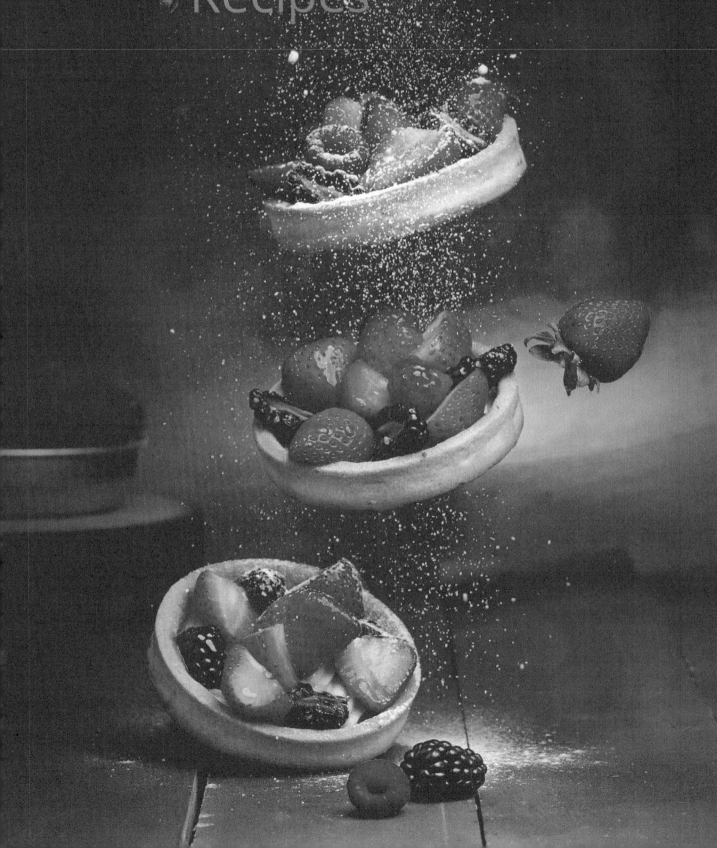

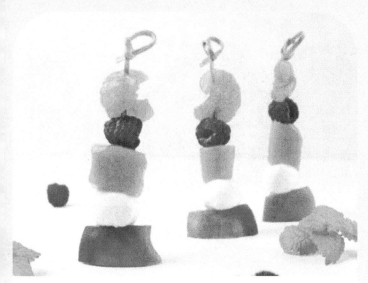

Apple and Peach Skewers (Italy)

Preparation time: 10 minutes
Servings: 4
Calories for serving: 140

Macronutrients

- Carbs:14 g
- Proteins: 2 g
- Fat: 0 g

Ingredients

- 1 big peach
- 2 apples
- 1 orange
- 2 mint leaves
- Olive oil to taste
- Salt and pepper to taste

Directions

1. First, peel the peach. Halve, remove the central stone, cut peach pulp and then cut it into cubes. Peel and remove the seed from the 2 apples, and wash and dry them.

2. Cut apples into cubes of the same size as the peach. Take a skewer and put first a cube of apple and then one of peach. Keep on this way until you have used up all the ingredients.

3. In the meantime, wash and dry the mint leaves. Put mint leaves in a bowl with oil, salt, and pepper and mix well.

4. Sprinkle the skewers with the mint emulsion, put them on serving plates and serve.

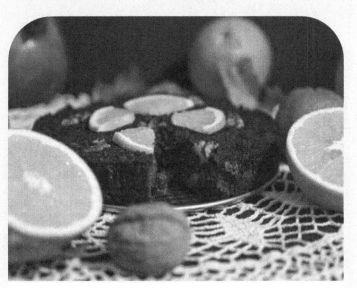

Almond Cocoa and Orange Pie (Italy)

Preparation time: 15 minutes
Cooking time: 40 minutes
Servings: 4
Calories for serving: 350

Macronutrients

- Carbs:29 g
- Proteins: 10 g
- Fat: 11 g

Ingredients

- 4 tbsp almond flour
- 2 tbsp sugar-free cocoa powder
- 4 tbsp almond milk
- 1 tbsp honey
- ½ tsp baking powder
- ½ tsp cinnamon
- 1 pinch salt
- 1 tbsp olive oil
- 2 tsp orange juice

Directions

1. Start by preparing the pie dough. In a bowl, combine all the dry ingredients: almond flour, baking soda, cocoa, cinnamon, and salt.

2. In a second bowl, combine now the liquid ingredients: olive oil, honey, almond milk, and orange juice. After that, combine the liquid and dry ingredients and mix well.

3. Line a baking pan with parchment paper and pour the cake dough.

4. Bake at 385°F in a static oven for 35/40 minutes, or until the cake is cooked and the surface is golden.

5. Remove from the oven and let the almond and cocoa cake cool before serving.

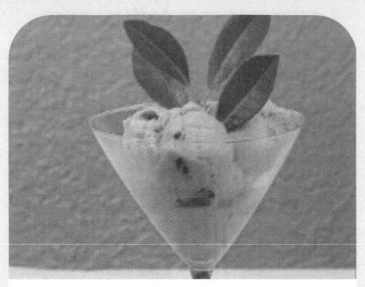

Cinnamon and Tangerine Sorbet (Italy)

Preparation time: 15 minutes
Servings: 4
Calories for serving: 70

Macronutrients

- Carbs: 9 g
- Proteins: 1 g
- Fat: 0 g

Ingredients

- 6 tangerines
- 1 tbsp ground cinnamon
- 2 tbsp honey
- 1 cup ice

Directions

1. First, peel the tangerines and remove only the pulp. Wash the zest and keep it aside.

2. Put the tangerines pulp, cinnamon, and honey in the blender glass.

3. Blend all ingredients at high speed for one minute.

4. Now add the ice and blend until you will obtain a homogeneous mixture.

5. Put the tangerine and cinnamon sorbet in the glasses, decorate with the tangerine zest and serve.

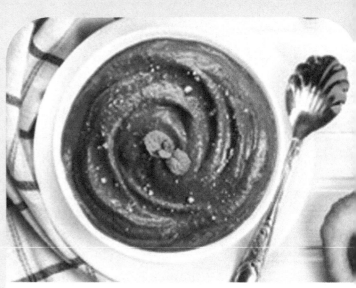

Coconut Pistachio and Cocoa Pudding (Italy)

Preparation time: 5 minutes
Cooking time: 5 minutes
Servings: 4
Calories for serving: 190

Macronutrients

- Carbs: 13 g
- Proteins: 6 g
- Fat: 5 g

Ingredients

- ½ cup and 2 tbsp coconut flour
- ½ cup water
- 2 tbsp milk
- 2 tbsp yogurt
- 2 tbsp sugar-free cocoa
- 1 tsp honey
- 2 tbsp chopped pistachios

Directions

1. First, put the yogurt in a microwave-safe bowl.

2. After that add coconut flour, water, milk, and cocoa powder.

3. Microwave for 45/50 seconds.

4. Then add coconut flour and honey and microwave for another 25–30 seconds.

5. Meanwhile, chop finely 2 tablespoons of pistachios. Serve pudding with a topping of chopped pistachios.

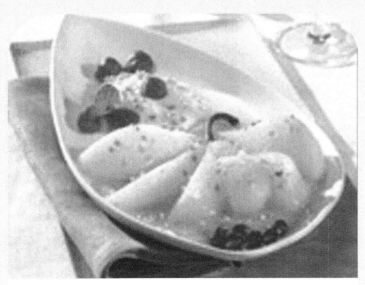

Hazelnut and Coconut Pear (Italy)

Preparation time: 15 minutes
Cooking time: 30 minutes
Servings: 4
Calories for serving: 200

Macronutrients

- Carbs: 14 g
- Proteins: 9 g
- Fat: 3 g

Ingredients

- 4 pears
- 4 tbsp melted coconut oil
- 2 tbsp powdered stevia
- 4 tbsp chopped hazelnuts
- 2 tbsp coconut flour
- Salt to taste

Directions

1. First, shell the pears, cut them in half, and remove the seeds, scooping each half pear very lightly with a teaspoon.

2. Oil a baking dish and arrange the pears, with the rounded part resting on the bottom of the container. Put the melted coconut olive oil in a bowl, together with the stevia, coconut flour, and a pinch of salt. Work the ingredients for a long time, until you get a soft, scent, and fluffy cream.

3. Chop the hazelnuts and add them to the coconut cream.

4. Now, divide the coconut and hazelnut mixture into eight parts and distribute it into the apple halves. Place in the oven at 390°F and cook for 25–30 minutes.

5. Take the pears, when cooked, out of the oven and let cool, then serve.

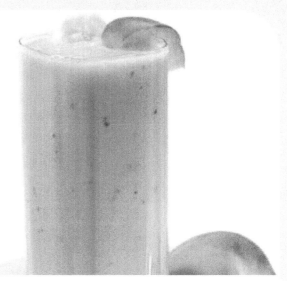

Peach and Apple Juice Shake (Italy)

Preparation time: 5 minutes
Cooking time: 5 minutes
Servings: 4
Calories for serving: 100

Macronutrients

- Carbs: 10 g
- Proteins: 2 g
- Fat: 1 g

Ingredients

- 2 peaches
- 2 cups unsweetened almond milk
- 4 ice cubes
- 2 tbsp fresh apple juice
- 1 tsp liquid stevia
- 1 tsp vanilla extract

Directions

1. First, peel and wash both peaches, remove the stone, and then cut them into pieces.

2. Put the peach pieces in the blender glass. Add the almond milk, vanilla, and stevia.

3. Turn on the blender and blend everything at maximum speed for one minute.

4. Now add the ice cubes and fresh apple juice and blend again until you get a thick and homogeneous mixture.

5. Transfer the shake into the glasses, add the straws and serve your peach shake.

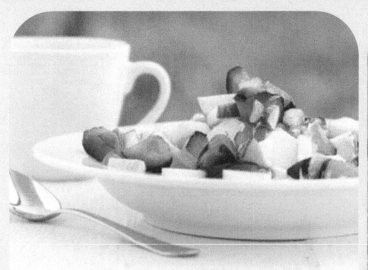

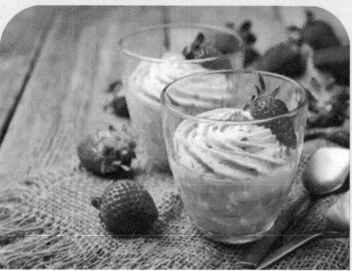

Plums and Lime Cinnamon Salad (Italy)

Preparation time: 30 minutes
Servings: 4
Calories for serving: 180

Macronutrients

- Carbs: 14 g
- Proteins: 5 g
- Fat: 6 g

Ingredients

- 2 plums
- 2 limes
- 2 tbsp sliced almonds
- 1 tsp cinnamon powder

Directions

1. First, wash the plums, remove the central stone, and then cut it into cubes.

2. Put plums in a large bowl and season with the lime juice. Add the sliced almonds too.

3. Sprinkle your salad with cinnamon, leave to flavor for 30 minutes and then put the fruit salad in serving bowls and serve your dessert.

Stracchino Strawberry and Vanilla Mousse (Italy)

Preparation time: 15 minutes
Cooking time: 20 minutes
Servings: 4
Calories for serving: 120

Macronutrients

- Carbs: 4 g
- Proteins: 18 g
- Fat: 2 g

Ingredients

- 1 cup and half of fresh stracchino cheese
- 1 tbsp vanilla powder
- 1 cup chopped strawberries
- 1 tsp stevia

Directions

1. Wash and dry the strawberries, then chop. Put strawberries and a glass of water in the saucepan and cook them with the stevia until you have obtained a sort of syrup.

2. Put the stracchino in a bowl and add the vanilla.

3. Stir and mix well and then add the strawberry syrup.

4. With the help of a manual whisk, combine the ingredients until you have obtained a smooth and compact mixture.

5. Put the stracchino mousse in the glasses and keep it in the fridge until you need to serve it.

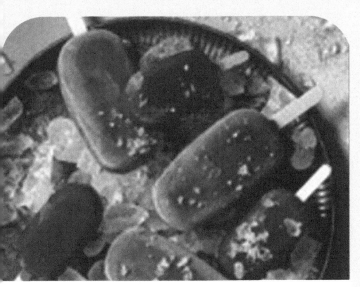

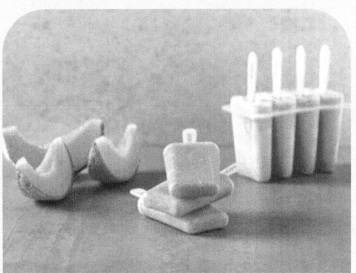

Vanilla and Sour Cherries Ice Cream (Italy)

Preparation time: 10 minutes
Rest time: 4 hours in the freezer
Servings: 4
Calories for serving: 150

Macronutrients

- Carbs:12 g
- Proteins: 5 g
- Fat: 6 g

Ingredients

- 2 cups pitted sour cherries
- ¼ cup skimmed milk
- 4 tbsp low sugar whipped cream
- 2 tbsp powdered stevia
- 1 tsp honey
- 1 tbsp vanilla extract

Directions

1. First, quickly rinse the pitted sour cherries in cold water, drain and lay them out to dry on a kitchen paper towel.

2. Blend the skimmed milk with the sour cherries, honey, and stevia in a blender until the mixture is homogeneous. Add the vanilla extract and mix and pour the mixture into the ice cream molds.

3. Place the stick in the center and let freeze your ice cream for at least 4 hours.

4. Turn out the sour cherries and vanilla ice cream and serve.

Watermelon, Ginger, and Orange Ice Cream

Preparation time: 15 minutes
Rest time: 2 hours in the freezer
Servings: 4
Calories for serving: 170

Macronutrients

- Carbs:15 g
- Proteins: 2 g
- Fat: 3 g

Ingredients

- 10 oz watermelon pulp (without seeds)
- 1 blood orange
- 1 cup sugar-free vegetable milk
- 1 tbsp powdered ginger
- 2 tbsp honey

Directions

1. First, remove the seeds from the watermelon and wash it. Cut watermelon pulp into pieces. Put the watermelon piece in the blender glass.

2. Add the vegetable milk and blend the ingredients at medium speed until you get a smooth and homogeneous mixture.

3. Add the honey, ginger, and juice of the blood orange. Keep on blending for another minute so that all the ingredients are well blended.

4. Put the obtained mixture in a container and put it in the freezer for an hour. Then transfer everything to the ice cream maker following the times indicated in the ice cream maker to prepare the ice cream.

5. Once it's ready, put the watermelon and orange ice cream back in the freezer to harden it, and then serve it.

Bonus Chapter: 21 Tips for Burning Excess Fat

Being overweight and obesity are two disabling physical conditions both physically and aesthetically. These are two limiting conditions for the life of people who suffer from these eating disorders as well as causing serious diseases, including chronic ones, for a long time.

Starting to change lifestyle and eating styles is essential to counter these two conditions. Although it is not an easy path to follow, especially at the beginning, patience, dedication and goodwill are the best weapons to face a period of change, at the end of which you will be able to appreciate the numerous benefits, both for health and for physical fitness.

Below you will find 21 useful tips to not only reduce body weight but also to transform fat mass, and therefore excess fat, into lean mass.

- **Tip 1 Include unsaturated fats in your diet and permanently eliminate saturated fats**

Unsaturated fats take a long time to digest and empty the stomach, thereby reducing appetite and hunger. One study found that the Mediterranean diet rich in unsaturated fatty acids from nuts and olive oil carries a lower risk of gaining weight than a calorie-restricted diet. In any case, even unsaturated fats should be consumed moderately, as they are always fat and consequently have a high caloric intake.

- **Tip 2 include foods that are high in fiber in your diet**

The fibers help the body absorb excess sugars during meals and being water-soluble they absorb a lot of water and move slowly through the intestinal tract, prolonging the sense of satiety over time. Eating foods with a high fiber content not only helps you lose weight but also helps to dispose of excess fat.

- **Tip 3 Eat nutrient-rich foods**

Eat a diet rich in micronutrients. This means eating a varied diet that includes all types of foods, mainly fruit, and vegetables. Many are fundamental in the metabolism of fats and therefore for the decrease of fat mass from the belly. They are also important for your overall health; they give you a lot of energy to use daily or during training.

- **Tip 4 drink only healthy drinks with no added sugar**

Permanently eliminating the consumption of carbonated and sugary drinks from your eating habits will help you lose fat and weight faster. Alcoholic beverages are also contained in this list. Alcohol also has a high-calorie content and, if consumed excessively or as a habit, leads to rapid weight gain.

- **Tip 5 Cut back on refined carbohydrate consumption**

Refined carbohydrates are both low in fiber and low in essential nutrients.

Furthermore, refined carbohydrates tend to have a high glycemic index, leading to sudden spikes in blood glucose levels and, consequently, also to a decrease in the sense of satiety. High consumption of refined carbohydrates also leads to a greater development of abdominal fat, also favoring the onset of some diseases.

- **Tip 6 Increase the iron intake**

Iron is one of the essential elements for carrying out various vital functions within the body. It is essential for the proper functioning of the thyroid, responsible for the secretion of hormones that regulate metabolism.

Increasing the intake of iron, through food or dietary supplements, allows the metabolism to work more effectively, as well as fight fatigue.

- **Tip 7 Never skip breakfast**

When you wake up in the morning, you have probably spent around 8 hours fasting and are therefore low on fuel. Skipping breakfast can cause your basal metabolic rate to drop by about 40%. So, skipping breakfast is bad for both health and fat loss. The ideal is to have a healthy and abundant breakfast that will avoid glycemic peaks during the day and will prevent you from overeating at lunch.

- **Tip 8 Avoid eating cereals in the early morning**

Do you like having milk and cereals for breakfast? In this case, you must be aware that these foods are high in sugar and therefore are not ideal if you want to lose weight and body fat. If you really can't give up cereals, then choose oats. In fact, they are rich in protein and have a satiating effect that allows you to eat less during the day.

- **Tip 9 Eat at least 3–5 servings of fruit and vegetables a day**

Fruits and vegetables contain fiber and take longer to digest. In addition, the fibers contained in fruits and vegetables can decrease the number of calories that the body absorbs and increase the sense of satiety.

- **Tip 10 Avoid snacking after dinner**

Most after-dinner snacks usually take place in an almost unconscious form. By skipping these snacks, you can cut other calories. In addition, going to bed knowing that you have eaten well will give you the energy to start over well with an excellent breakfast and continue on the path of weight loss and excess fat loss.

- **Tip 11 Don't dine too late in the evening**

Our digestive system needs some time to burn the evening meal. Therefore, it is advisable not to dine too late, as the closer to sleep we take in calories, the less time our body will have to consume them.

- **Tip 12 Categorically abolishes junk food**

Junk food is a type of food rich in fats, including trans ones, which are harmful to the waist and health because they favor the increase of adipose tissue. These foods are often eaten as a snack: a good strategy for decreasing weight and body fat is to opt for healthier and more nutritious snacks.

- **Tip 13 Include fatty fish rich in omega-3 and omega-6 in your diet**

Fatty fish are incredibly healthy and helpful in lowering blood fat levels. They are rich in high-quality proteins and omega-3 fats that protect you from diseases, especially those of cardiovascular origin.

Some evidence suggests that these omega-3 fats help reduce visceral fat.

Studies in some adults with fatty liver show that fish oil supplements can significantly reduce liver fat and abdominal fat.

- **Tip 14 Take probiotics**

Probiotics are good bacteria that promote the proper functioning of the intestinal tract. Recent studies have shown that integrating probiotic-rich foods into one's diet resulted in a large increase in both weight loss and body fat.

- **Tip 15 Drink at least two liters of water a day**

Water is the source of life. Staying well hydrated is therefore essential. In addition, it is possible to cut calories by replacing water with other caloric drinks. Drinking more water will improve your body's ability to process ingested food and will help keep your core body temperature low during workouts, reducing the perception of exertion and avoiding confusing thirst with feeling hungry.

- **Tip 16 Drink more coffee**

Coffee is a very useful substance and without sugar is zero calories, which, by stimulating the central nervous system, increases both the metabolism and the disposal of fatty acids. In addition, coffee improves the elimination of fats during aerobic exercise.

- **Tip 17 Get moving by practicing cardio**

Cardio activities are a series of aerobic exercises that are done to specifically train the body and lungs.

Adding this type of activity to a daily training routine, followed by a healthy diet, allows you to burn fat quickly and in large quantities. To reduce fat, it is advisable to practice between 150 and 300 minutes of aerobic exercise per week, then 20–40 minutes per day, at a moderate or sustained level.

- **Tip 18 Start walking or running**

Walking briskly or running for 30 minutes every day will help you not only feel fit but also deflate your prominent abdomen by promoting intestinal transit of food and improving digestion. This way you will lose excess weight and fat.

- **Tip 19 Start exercising to improve muscle strength**

To start reducing body fat and losing weight, strength exercises are extremely useful, such as weightlifting, which also allows you to increase muscle mass.

A study has shown that muscle strength training allows you to reduce intra-abdominal fat, a very dangerous type of fat because it accumulates around the internal organs, in people suffering from metabolic syndromes.

Another study found that people who did 12-week strength training paired with aerobic exercise reduced body fat more effectively than those who did only aerobic exercise.

In addition, this type of training allows you to develop and preserve lean mass, allowing you to increase the number of calories burned when the body is at rest.

- **Tip 20 Try to Sleep More**

Sleeping properly will help you increase weight and body fat loss. A tip for getting adequate sleep is to try to go to bed earlier and wake up a little later than usual.

Studies of people who suffered from sleep disorders and slept less than 6 hours a night showed that they were more likely to gain weight and increase body fat levels.

If you want to eliminate excess fat, then try to sleep at least 7 hours a night.

- **Tip 21 Try to Reduce Stress**

Stress releases a hormone called cortisol in our bodies. Excessive levels of cortisol can lead to weight gain, particularly visceral belly weight. What is the best way to decrease stress levels? Practicing regular relaxation techniques, such as deep breathing and meditation, to stay calm and reduce stress levels seem like a small thing, and instead, according to science, they are a great help against excess cortisol and its side effects.

FAQ

1. Is it true that with the Mediterranean diet you stuff yourself with bread and pasta?

Those who pass off the colossal eating of spaghetti with tomato as a Mediterranean diet are misleading.

In the Guidelines for a healthy Mediterranean diet, the standard serving of pasta, bread, or rice for a 1500 kcal diet is 80 grams, once a day.

2. Is it necessary to dissociate carbohydrates from proteins?

The dissociated diet does not make sense, even for the mere fact that pasta or even fruit have a protein share. Not only that: carbohydrates and proteins are supported. Insulin, the hormone produced by the pancreas to regulate the presence of glucose in the blood, favors the use of amino acids, the building blocks of proteins, for protein synthesis.

In addition, protein burns calories better than carbohydrates during digestion and gives a sense of satiety.

3. Is the Mediterranean diet a carnivorous food model?

The Mediterranean diet is considered an omnivorous model. The Mediterranean diet indeed includes animal proteins, none excluded, but it is mainly a vegetable type of diet, with fruit, vegetables in abundance, legumes, and cereals.

4. Is it a difficult diet to follow?

The Mediterranean diet ranked first in the easiest-to-follow diets category, according to US News & World Report.

Simplicity is given by various factors: it does not prohibit entire food groups, there are hundreds of recipes to be made in a few minutes and with few ingredients and you can also eat away from home by easily finding the dishes to compose a menu in perfect Mediterranean style.

5. Is it an expensive diet?

It is certainly not an inexpensive way of eating but spending a few more bucks to buy healthy foods is certainly convenient on an aesthetic and organic level.

6. Is the Mediterranean diet the choice of proper nutrition?

The Mediterranean diet is considered a complete and balanced eating style, and when it comes to proper nutrition we are inspired by this model. In fact, it has been shown that it guarantees a good state of nutrition (and therefore of health), preventing cardiovascular diseases.

7. What are the basic principles of the Mediterranean diet?

The principles of the Mediterranean diet are greater consumption of cereals, preferably whole grains, a source of complex carbohydrates and fiber, with a decrease in the consumption of simple carbohydrates and refined sugars; reduction of saturated fats, and consumption of olive oil, a precious source of mono and polyunsaturated fats; greater consumption of proteins of vegetable origin, or legumes; high intake of fruits and vegetables, sources of dietary fiber and vitamins; consume white meats more than red meats; active and healthy lifestyle.

8. Why is it called the Mediterranean diet?

Because it is a food model based on the eating and living habits of the people bordering the Mediterranean Sea.

9. Will I suffer from hunger following the Mediterranean diet?

No, absolutely. Because while it is true that you are cutting down on junk food and sugars, they will be replaced by healthier, lower calorie, and high-satiating foods such as fruits and vegetables.

10. Why should I follow a Mediterranean-style diet?

Because it is a healthy and not very restrictive diet. In fact, thanks to the variety of foods included in the diet, it turns out to be a healthy and complete eating style.

11. Is the Mediterranean diet another trendy diet that doesn't give any results?

It must be specified that the Mediterranean diet is not a diet that is followed for a few weeks or months, but a lifestyle, a food style that must be followed throughout life.

12. Does the Mediterranean diet involve the consumption of strange or hard-to-find foods?

The foods included in the Mediterranean diet are readily available and can also be found in local markets or supermarkets.

13. Can I eat sweets if I follow the Mediterranean diet?

Desserts should be avoided and consumed occasionally and only on special occasions. In addition, it would be better to consume homemade desserts and avoid those of industrial origin or preserved.

14. Is it true that it is possible to lose weight with the Mediterranean diet?

Although it was not born as a diet aimed at weight loss, following a Mediterranean diet it is also possible to lose a good amount of excess weight.

15. Can I drink wine if I follow a Mediterranean diet?

You can drink wine but in moderation. In fact, it is allowed to drink a glass of wine either at lunch or dinner.

16. Do I have to keep track of calories if I follow the Mediterranean diet?

It is not necessary to count calories or keep a food diary if you follow this diet. Cutting carbohydrates and reducing fat already provide a lower-than-normal calorie intake.

17. Can the Mediterranean diet be followed by those suffering from diabetes?

Yes, the Mediterranean diet is ideal for those suffering from diabetes, especially for those suffering from type 2 diabetes. This is possible thanks to the increase in the intake of vegetables and foods rich in fiber and the decrease in the intake of unsaturated fats and sugar-rich, prepackaged foods.

18. Does the Mediterranean diet lower cholesterol levels?

Yes, the Mediterranean diet lowers cholesterol levels. Thanks to the contribution of antioxidants and fibers, the levels of LDL cholesterol or bad cholesterol go down and the levels of HDL cholesterol, or good cholesterol, increase.

19. Can the Mediterranean diet be followed by vegans/vegetarians?

The Mediterranean diet has the highest basic consumption of vegetables and fruit; therefore, yes, it is perfect for those who follow vegan and vegetarian diets. Animal proteins can then be easily replaced by vegetable ones.

20. Does the Mediterranean diet involve the consumption of smoothies?

Yes, in the Mediterranean diet you can drink fruit smoothies with peace of mind. However, the only thing you need to keep in mind is not to overdo it with sugars. In fact, in order not to exceed it, just do not add granulated sugar and replace it with honey and use low-sugar milk.

30 Days Meal Plans

Below you will find examples of meal plans to follow for 30 days. Meal plans are generic and are all 1600 calories. You will find in the meal plan the foods with the daily quantities that you can replace with the recipes indicated in the previous chapters

	Breakfast	Lunch	Dinner	Calories
Day 1	1 cup semi-skimmed milk + 3.5 oz fresh seasonal fruit	1 soup + 1 salad	5.2 oz chicken + 1 salad + 1.7 oz wholemeal bread	1600
Day 2	Natural white yogurt + 1 oz whole grains + 1 glass unsweetened fruit juice	1 salad + 7 oz mackerel	80 oz pasta + 7 oz zucchinis + 5.2 oz turkey	1600
Day 3	1 smoothie	1 soup + 1.7 oz wholemeal bread + 1 salad	7 oz tuna + 7 oz vegetables + 1.7 oz wholemeal bread	1600
Day 4	1 omelet + 3.5 oz fresh seasonal fruit	2.4 oz rice + 1 salad	5.2 oz turkey + 7 oz potatoes	1600
Day 5	1 cup partially skimmed cow's milk + 2 wholemeal rusks + citrus jam with no added sugar	2.4 oz di pasta + 1 salad	7 oz cod + 7 oz vegetables + 1.7 oz wholemeal bread	1600

Day 6	1 omelet+ 3.5 oz fresh seasonal fruit	4.2 oz beef + 1 salad + 1.7 oz wholemeal bread	1 fish soup 7 oz vegetables	1600
Day 7	1 smoothie + 2 wholemeal rusks with honey	2.4 oz pasta + 1 salad	1 vegetable soup + 5.2 oz chicken + 1.7 oz wholemeal bread	1600
Day 8	1 cup semi-skimmed milk + 2 wholemeal rusks 2 tbsp jam with no added sugar	7 oz salmon+ 1 salad + 1.7 oz wholemeal bread	1 stew + 1 vegetable salad + 1.7 oz wholemeal bread	1600
Day 9	2 eggs + 3.5 oz fresh seasonal fruit	2.4 oz rice + 7 oz mushroom	7 oz octopus + 7 oz vegetables + 1.7 oz wholemeal bread	1600
Day 10	1 smoothie + 2 wholemeal biscuits	7 oz sea bass + 7 oz potatoes	2.8 oz lentils+ 1 salad	1600
Day 11	1 cup Greek yogurt+ 1.7 oz berries	2.8 oz rice+ 7 oz salmon+ 7 oz vegetables	4.2 oz pork+ 7 oz vegetables	1600
Day 12	1 omelet + 3.5 oz vegetables	2.8 oz chickpeas + 5.2 oz vegetables + 3.5 oz fruit	5.2 oz beef + 7 oz spinach + 1.7 oz wholemeal bread	1600

Day 13	1 cup green tea + 1 small piece of 85% dark chocolate + 5.2 oz fresh seasonal fruit	2.4 oz pasta + 7 oz peppers	7 oz calamari + 7 oz potatoes	1600
Day 14	½ cup low-fat plain yogurt with no added sugar + 5.2 oz strawberries	2.8 oz beans + 7 oz cod	7 oz tuna + 1 salad + 1.7 oz wholemeal bread	1600
Day 15	½ cup semi-skimmed milk + 2 wholemeal rusks + 2 tsp jam with no added sugar + 5 dry walnuts	7–8 oz sea bream + 1 salad + 1.7 oz wholemeal bread	1 vegetable soup + 5.2 oz chicken + 1.7 oz wholemeal bread	1600
Day 16	1 cup herbal tea + 1.7 oz wholemeal rye bread + 1 tbsp almond cream + 1 banana	1 stew + 1 salad + 1.7 oz wholemeal bread	3.5 oz fresh cheese 7 oz vegetables + 1.7 oz wholemeal bread	1600
Day 17	1 omelet + 1 peach	5.2 oz turkey + 7 oz vegetables + 1.7 oz wholemeal bread	2.4 oz rice + 7 oz shrimp	1600

Day 18	4.4 oz low-fat white yogurt with no added sugar + 5.2 oz fresh seasonal fruit	5.2 oz chicken + 7 oz potatoes + 3.5 oz vegetables	7 oz salmon + 7 oz vegetables + 1.7 oz wholemeal bread	1600
Day 19	1 cup herbal tea + 1 omelet	7 oz sea bass + 7 oz vegetables + 1.7 oz wholemeal bread	3.5 oz feta cheese + 1 salad + 1 oz wholemeal bread	1600
Day 20	1 cup Greek yogurt + 3.5 oz strawberries	2.1 oz lentils + 3.5 oz chicken + 1 vegetable salad	7 oz sea bream + 1 salad + 1.7 oz wholemeal bread	1600
Day 21	1 cup semi-skimmed milk, 2 oz wholemeal rusks, 2 tbsp jam with no added sugar	2.4 oz pasta+ 7 oz tuna +7 oz peppers	7 oz cod + 1 salad + 1.7 oz wholemeal bread	1600
Day 22	1 omelet + 7 oz fresh seasonal fruit	5.2 oz lamb + 7 oz vegetables	3.5 oz fresh cheese + 7 oz vegetables + 1.7 oz wholemeal bread	1600
Day 23	1 cup semi-skimmed milk 1 cup coffee 2 wholemeal biscuits	2.4 oz pasta +3.5 oz tuna + 7 oz vegetables	7 oz octopus + 1 salad + 1.7 oz wholemeal bread	1600
Day 24	1 smoothie + 2 wholemeal rusks	2.4 oz rice + 5.2 oz salmon + 7 oz vegetables	5.2 oz beef + 1 salad + 1 oz wholemeal bread	1600

	+0.7 oz 85% dark chocolate			
Day 25	1 glass fruit juice with no added sugar 1 omelet	2.8 oz cous cous+ 5.2 oz chicken+ 7 oz vegetables	7 oz mackerel + 7 oz potatoes + 1 peach	1600
Day 26	1 cup semi-skimmed milk 1 coffee + 3.5 oz fresh seasonal fruit	2.4 oz pasta +1 carrot salad +3.5 oz chicken	1 meat soup +1.7 oz wholemeal bread +7 oz vegetables	1600
Day 27	1 smoothie + 12 almonds + 1 wholemeal rusk	2.4 oz rice+ 7 oz mackerel+ 7 oz vegetables	5.2 oz pork + 1 salad + 1 oz wholemeal bread	1600
Day 28	1 cup semi-skimmed milk + 3.5 oz fresh seasonal fruit	1 stew +1 salad + 1.7 oz wholemeal bread	5.2 oz turkey + 7 oz vegetables + 1.7 oz wholemeal bread	1600
Day 29	4.4 oz low-fat white yogurt with no added sugar + 5.2 oz fresh seasonal fruit	2.8 oz rice+ 7 oz salmon + 7 oz vegetables	5.2 oz beef + 7 oz spinach + 1.7 oz wholemeal bread	1600
Day 30	1 cup green tea +1 small piece of 85% dark chocolate + 5.2 oz fresh seasonal fruit	2.4 oz pasta+ 7 oz tuna +7 oz peppers	2.1 oz lentils + 3.5 oz chicken + 1 vegetable salad	1600

Measurement Conversion Chart

DRY WEIGHTS

1/2 oz	1 tbsp	-	15 g
1 oz	2 tbsp	1/8 c	28 g
2 oz	4 tbsp	1/4 c	57 g
3 oz	6 tbsp	1/3 c	85 g
4 oz	8 tbsp	1/2 c	115 g
8 oz	16 tbsp	1 cup	227 g
12 oz	24 tbsp	1½ c	340 g
16 oz	32 tbsp	2 c	455 g

1 OZ = 28 GRAMS
1 LBS = 454 G
1 CUP = 227 G

1 TSP = 5 ML
1 TBSP = 15 ML
1 OZ = 30 ML
1 CUP = 237 ML
1 PINT = 473 ML (2 CUPS)
1 GALLON = 16 CUPS

LIQUID VOLUMES

1 oz	2 tbsp	1/8 c	30 ml
2 oz	4 tbsp	1/4 c	60 ml
2⅔ oz	6 tbsp	1/3 c	80 ml
4 oz	8 tbsp	1/2 c	120 ml
8 oz	16 tbsp	2/3 c	160 ml
12 oz	24 tbsp	3/4 c	177 ml
16 oz	32 tbsp	1 cup	237 ml
32 oz	64 tbsp	1½ c	470 ml
		2 c	950 ml

ABBREVIATIONS

tbsp = Tablespoon
tsp = Teaspoon
fl.oz - Fluid Ounce
c = cup
ml = Milliliter
lb = pound
F = Fahrenheit
C = Celsius
ml = Milliliter
g = grams
kg = kilogram
l = liter

BAKING PAN

9-inch (by 3") standard round pan = 12 cups
9-inch (by 2.5") springform pan = 10 cups
10-inch (by 4") tube pan = 16 cups
9-inch (by 3") bundt pan = 12 cups
9-inch (by 2") square pan = 10 cups
9 x 5 inch loaf pan = 8 cups

OVEN TEMP.

130 c = 250 F
165 c = 325 F
177 c = 350 F
190 c = 375 F
200 c = 400 F
220 c = 425 F

Conclusions

In this guide, you have found all the instructions to start following one of the most famous and healthy diets in the world. You have been offered daily plans to follow with their respective recipes so that you can better approach this new style, which is not just a healthy eating style to follow, but a real lifestyle.

If you want to start getting better, lose a few extra pounds, or avoid diseases related to well-being, the Mediterranean diet is the one for you. As you could understand from the guide, this diet is safe, not restrictive, and suitable for everyone.

In conclusion, we can certainly say that the Mediterranean diet is the best food approach known so far.

What is important to underline regarding the Mediterranean diet is the wonderful and huge variety of foods it includes and the carefree nature with which it is lived.

The real great and precious secret of the Mediterranean diet lies in its balance, which makes it tasty and varied, without unnecessary sacrifices.

Made in the USA
Coppell, TX
14 December 2022

89264585R00046